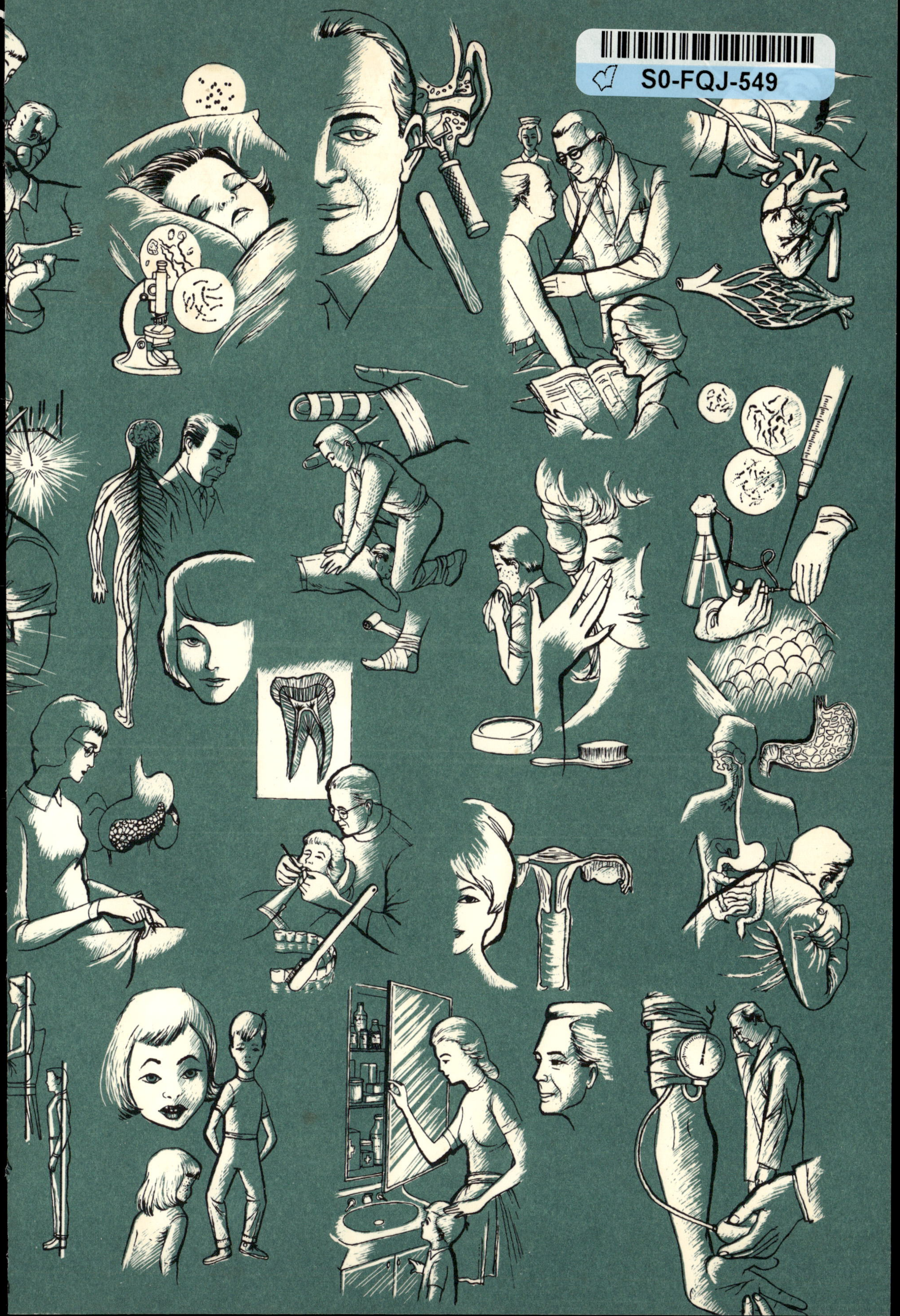

VOLUME **3**

CANCER
TO
CONTUSION

This volume is unified and cross
indexed to consulting discussions on
CANCER
Pages 319-354

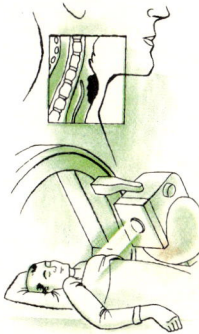

the *New* illustrated

Medical and

Health

Encyclopedia

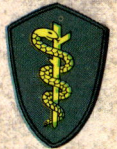

edited by

MORRIS FISHBEIN, M.D.

**With the Collaboration
of 60 Leading Specialists in
Medicine and Surgery**

H. S. STUTTMAN CO., Inc. Publishers
New York 16, N. Y.

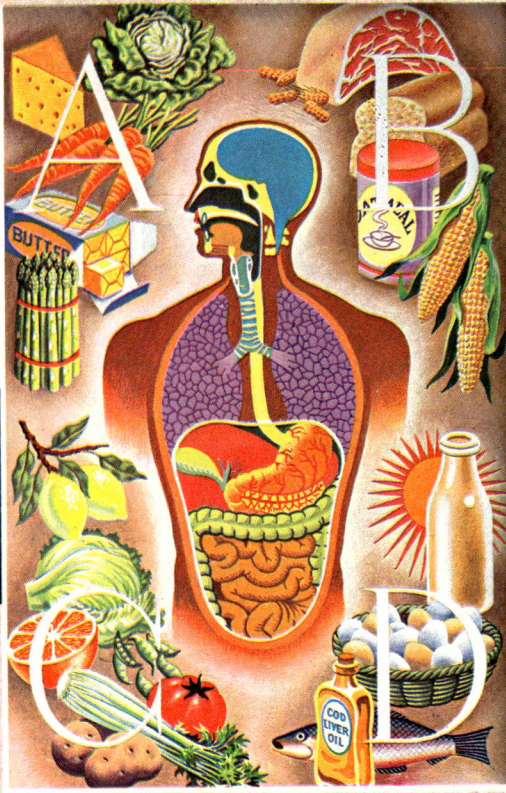

PICTORIAL FEATURE
Your Digestive System

Pages 325-332

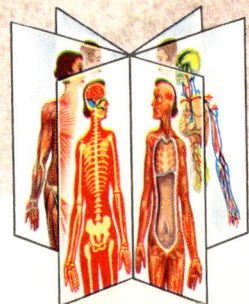

Litho in U.S.A.

Where Cancer Strikes

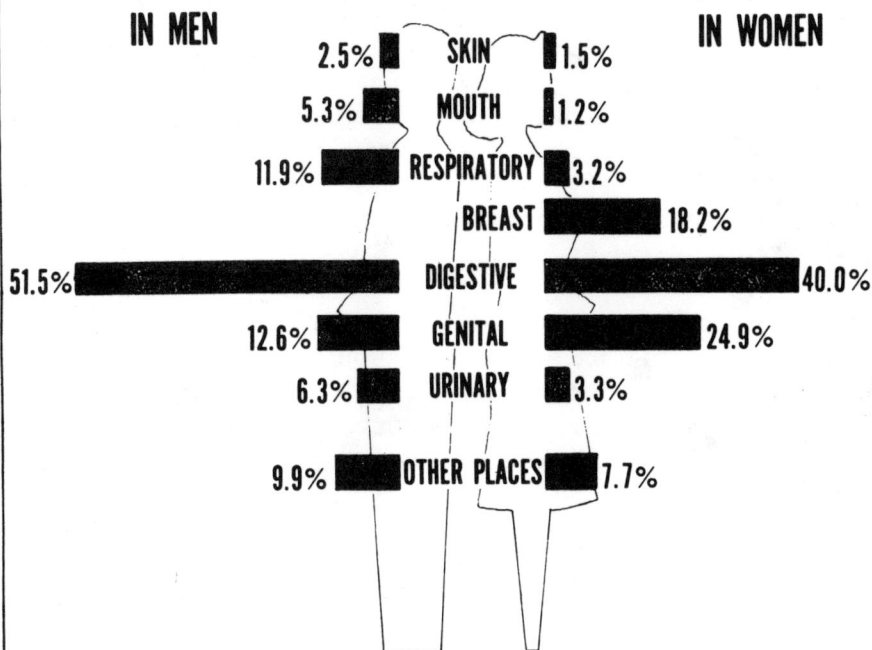

IN MEN		IN WOMEN
2.5%	SKIN	1.5%
5.3%	MOUTH	1.2%
11.9%	RESPIRATORY	3.2%
	BREAST	18.2%
51.5%	DIGESTIVE	40.0%
12.6%	GENITAL	24.9%
6.3%	URINARY	3.3%
9.9%	OTHER PLACES	7.7%

Charts by Graphics Institute, N.Y.C.

CANCER, a disease characterized by abnormal and often unpredictable growth of cells. Cancerous growths are also disposed to invade normal healthy tissues which can be destroyed or even replaced by their wild growth. Nerves may be affected, causing pain; blood vessels may be broken open by the invading growth, causing hemorrhage; and structures such as lung tissues, the arteries, kidneys, or bladder may be obstructed by infiltration of cancer tissue. Every part of the body is susceptible to cancerous growths, though some organs, such as stomach, bowel, lung, and the sexual organs, seem more frequently involved.

Accumulations of rapidly growing cells may form a lump known as a tumor, but not all tumors are cancerous or dangerous. Many, such as fibromas, clumps of scar-type tissue; adenomas, clumps of harmless glandular tissue; warts, fatty tumors, or lipomas do not invade normal tissue and do not lead to serious consequences. They are benign or harmless growths or tumors. Groups of cells which invade normal tissue and destroy healthy cells are malignant. Growth may be rapid or slow, but usually is progressive; that is, the cancers do not stop growing once they originate.

Some cancers remain in one location; others tend to spread through the blood stream or lymphatic stream throughout the body. These "pilgrim-type" growths, metastases, in general represent a more serious type of cancer.

The exact cause of cancer is unknown. Some scientists believe that persons are born with abnormal cells and that these remain quiescent throughout life or until some factor starts them growing. Others believe that chronic irritation of a certain group of cells may lead to cancerous changes. Cancer of the lip is common in pipe smokers and lung cancer in cigarette smokers. Some specialists feel that irritation from the sun may lead to skin cancers, common in farmers and outdoor workers. Chemicals also may induce cancer. The sex hormones are related to cancer development, especially of the breast or reproductive system. Because wives of circumcised men rarely develop cancer of the cervix, some experts believe that the uncircumcised male may harbor a cancer-producing secretion under the foreskin. A relationship may exist between failure to breast feed and breast cancer. Heredity is probably significant, but just how is not yet known. Cancer is probably not contagious; nevertheless, experiments utilizing our knowledge of viruses are being made to confirm this.

Kinds of cancer. Doctors classify cancer according to many factors: the type of tissue involved; the speed of its growth; the portion of the body involved; and sometimes even according to the chemical changes that take place within the tumor.

Some cancers are easily seen or felt, such as breast and skin cancers; some can be detected or suspected by rectal or vaginal examination and by introduction of instruments into the stomach; some by x-ray, by blood or urine tests, and by other techniques.

Certain cancers—for instance, breast cancers—are found predominantly in women; lung and mouth cancers are more common in men.

The symptoms of early cancers are often barely noticeable; therefore, everyone should have a complete and thorough medical checkup at least once a year, and oftener if abnormal symptoms occur. Lives are needlessly lost because cancer is diagnosed much too late for the doctor to achieve successful treatment. Often the symptoms are caused by a harmless condition, but delay in treatment can be hazardous.

Any of the following symptoms should be checked promptly by a competent physician.

Mouth. Any sore in the mouth, or anywhere for that matter, that lasts more than a few days without healing should be reported.

Larynx. Hoarseness that persists for more than a week, and for three weeks at the most, should be suspected. By examination of the vocal cords, the doctor can determine whether or not they are inflamed or irritated, or affected by tumors of a benign or malignant nature. Removal of the growths and examination of the specimen under the microscope will aid in making the diagnosis.

Breast. Any discomfort, pain, thickening, dimpling, or lump in a breast of a man or woman that does not disappear within a week, and any discharge from the nipple, bloody or otherwise, demands immediate attention. Delay can be perilous. If the doctor demands surgical removal of the lump for expert examination, this should be done without delay as only by microscopic examination of tissue can definite diagnosis be made.

Stomach. Stomach cancer seldom causes pain. Ordinarily early signs include loss of appetite, diarrhea, appearance of black material in the stools, regurgitation, or difficulty in swallowing food. Generally these symptoms point to conditions less serious than cancer, and the doctor can make correct diagnosis by using x-ray and other techniques.

Female organs. Prolonged, irregular, or unusual bleeding, especially after the age of thirty-five or between periods, should always be investigated promptly.

New aids to cancer diagnosis. Cancer may be diagnosed in many different ways, some simple, others complicated. Most significant is a detailed history of the onset and nature of the patient's symptoms, followed by a thorough examination. When suspicious growths are noted on the skin, in the breasts, or within the reproductive organs, the doctor may take a piece of tissue for examination under the microscope. This is known as biopsy. The cancer cell, when viewed under the microscope, is different from the normal cell. In some cases, changes in the cells may be difficult to detect, even by experts.

Among the most recent medical discoveries is the Papanicolaou test for cancer. In this test, scrapings taken from the surface of the cervix of the uterus or from the walls of the vagina are treated with certain chemicals. The tissues are then placed under the microscope, where careful examination can usually rule out or indicate the presence of early cancer changes. The test can be used on the sputum of presumed lung cancer, and also on stomach secretion when cancer in that organ is suspected.

Tissue from within the body can be removed for analysis by curettage, as in the uterus when the uterus wall is scraped. Investigation may be performed by bronchoscopy, in which a long tube is inserted into the lung structure to remove tissue; by gastroscopy, done with a stomach tube; or proctoscopy, in which a long telescope-like instrument is inserted into the rectum. These instruments used for detecting cancer are often provided with a light so that the operator can actually look into the organs.

X-ray is invaluable in detecting cancer. To aid in finding stomach or rectal cancer, barium, a white substance, is introduced into these organs and helps x-rays detect any tumors by outlining them. Occasionally substances may be injected into the blood stream which outline the kidneys or other organs.

Blood tests for the detection of cancer, except for cancer of the blood, are being studied extensively, but as yet none of the tests has been accepted.

Is cancer caused by a germ? Some scientists are inclined to feel that cancer may be caused by a virus, a form of living growth too small to be seen under the microscope. Already there seems to be evidence that certain

315

substances like viruses can cause cancers. A factor that passes through the mother's milk in mice has been found capable of causing cancer in other mice. However, this finding is not applicable to human beings.

Another technique that has aroused interest is the attempt to grow tumors in yolk sacs of developing chicks. Here certain viruses are grown and distinguished from one another. Success has been reported in growing transplants from breast cancer on yolk sacs of chick embryos. This may not prove that viruses cause cancer, but rather that cancer cells can grow on a suitable medium if transplanted. At present experiments are being conducted on human beings by inoculating volunteers with deadly cancer cells. The results may have far-reaching effects on our knowledge and treatment of cancer.

Hormones, particularly sex hormones, may stimulate cancer growth. These include the female hormone, estrogen, and the male hormone, testosterone. Estrogens in large amounts may stimulate growth of breast cancers while they may delay growth of male cancers, notably prostate cancers. The male hormone may actually help to stop the growth of female breast cancer, and conversely stimulate prostate cancer.

Is cancer hereditary? Studies on animals indicate that the tendency to develop cancer seems stronger in some families than in others, although there does not seem to be a true inheritance. In some families, cancer apparently will develop in certain circumstances. Therefore, when any cancer is common in one family, members of the family should avoid taking sex hormones and overexposure to x-rays or to other chemicals or irritants.

Cancer-stimulating substances are thought to include coal tars, x-rays, excessive exposure to the sun, viruses, and hormones. Mechanical irritation, such as tight girdles or collars and friction on a mole on the skin may be harmful. Rough teeth and improperly fitted dentures may, by causing irritation, lead to cancer of the mouth, as may pipe and cigarette smoking.

Cancer of the blood usually manifests itself by anemia, fatigue, loss of weight, and shortness of breath. The diagnosis is made by examining the blood and a specimen of tissue taken from the bone marrow.

Treatment. Surgery has always been one of the most effective ways to remove cancers. By the removal of localized growths, the patient may be completely cured. Approach to treatment may be varied, and may not, in some cases, even include surgery. X-ray, or radium treatment is employed successfully in many types of pelvic cancer. Chemical therapy includes hormone treatments of breast and prostate cancer, and also drug management of the leukemias, blood cancers. Often a combination of surgery, x-ray, and drugs is used.

Most exciting of recent approaches to treatment is the use of radioactive isotopes. The isotopes are chemicals having radioactivity combined with a chemical element. Since these chemicals are likely to go directly to one tissue of the body, they concentrate in that organ and destroy abnormal tissues there. Cancer of the thyroid has been successfully treated by using radioactive iodine. Iron, sodium, potassium, chlorine, bromine, calcium, strontium, sulphur, carbon, and hydrogen have all been subjected to experiments in controlling growths in various parts of the body. Radioactive phosphorus has also been applied externally to warts, moles, and other growths on the surface of the body, and in some instances with apparent success.

The nitrogen mustard chemicals, developed for use in warfare, have been helpful in destroying cancer cells of the blood. These drugs are used effectively in Hodgkin's disease, chronic leukemia, and in other forms of blood tumors.

Much remains to be learned about cancer, and much will depend on the cooperation of patients in promptly reporting to their doctor any suspicious signs. Regular yearly checkups aid in early detection of cancers.

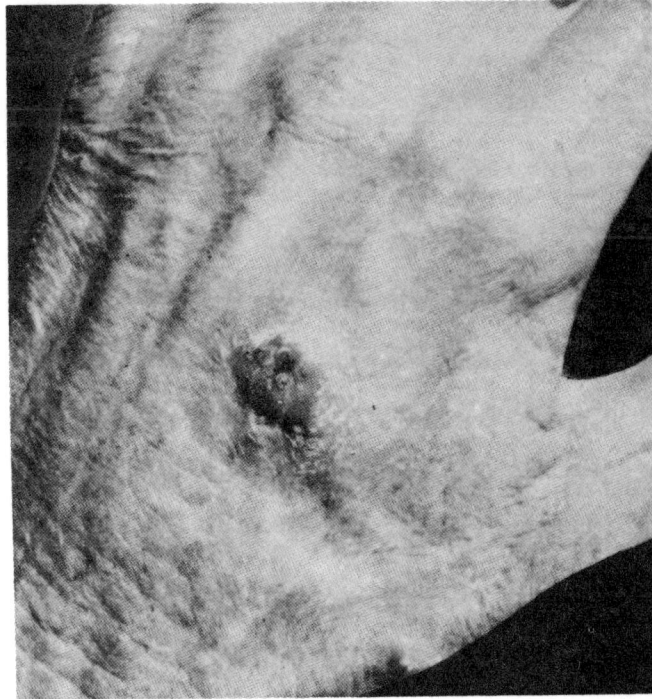

Skin Cancer — There are various types of skin cancer. To identify what type of cancer is affecting the hand, a piece of tissue will be removed for examination (biopsy). Laboratory tests and microscopic study reveal what kind of cells make up the tissue and thus the type of cancerous tumor present.

CANCER – causes: See article CANCER, page 320-21.

CANCER – children: See article CANCER, page 349-50.

CANCER – danger signals: See article CANCER, page 321-22.

CANCER – death rate: See article DISEASES OF THE HEART AND CIRCULATION, page 979.

CANCER – defined: See article CANCER, page 319.

CANCER – diagnosis: See article CANCER, page 320-22.

CANCER – diarrhea caused by: See article DIGESTION AND DIGESTIVE DISEASES, page 898.

CANCER – distribution: See article CANCER, page 320.

CANCER – drugs for: See article DRUGS AND THEIR USES, page 613-14.

CANCER – esophagus: See articles DIGESTION AND DIGESTIVE DISEASES, page 881; CANCER, pages 326, 335.

CANCER – gall bladder: See article DIGESTION AND DIGESTIVE DISEASES, pages 874, 876.

CANCER – gallstones: See article DIGESTION AND DIGESTIVE DISEASES, page 889.

CANCER – gastritis: See article DIGESTION AND DIGESTIVE DISEASES, page 883.

CANCER – genitals: See article SEX HYGIENE, page 1703-05.

CANCER – goiter: See article ENDOCRINOLOGY, page 682-83.

CANCER – heart disease more expensive in cost of human lives: See article DISEASES OF THE HEART AND CIRCULATION, page 978-79.

CANCER – hereditary factor: See article CANCER, pages 350, 352.

CANCER – hormones, importance of: See article CANCER, page 352-53.

CANCER – hypotension: See article BLOOD PRESSURE, page 265-66.

CANCER – incidence among women over forty: See article SEX HYGIENE, page 1703-04.

CANCER – intestinal obstruction: See article DIGESTION AND DIGESTIVE DISEASES, page 901.

CANCER – intestines: See article CANCER, page 336-39.

CANCER – keratoses: See article THE SKIN, pages 1767, 1769.

CANCER – lactic acid in stomach indicates: See article DIGESTION AND DIGESTIVE DISEASES, pages 872, 874.

CANCER – larynx: See article CANCER, pages 325-26, 335.

CANCER – lip: See article CANCER, page 324-26.

CANCER – lung: See article CANCER, page 343-46.

CANCER – lymph nodes spread: See article CANCER, page 335-36.

CANCER – mouth: See article CANCER, page 324-26.

CANCER – old age: See article OLD AGE, page 914-15.

CANCER – periodic health checkup important in detecting: See article CANCER, page 354.

CANCER – platelet count decreased: See article THE BLOOD AND ITS DISEASES, page 1046.

CANCER – prostate: See articles SEX HYGIENE, page 1704-05; CANCER, page 346-48; OLD AGE, page 914-15.

CANCER – quacks: See article CANCER, page 323-24.

CANCER – radiant energy may cause: See article OCCUPATION AND HEALTH, page 1372.

CANCER – research: See article CANCER, pages 350, 352-53.

CANCER – senile freckles may result in: See article THE SKIN, page 1778.

CANCER – signs and symptoms: See article CANCER, pages 323-26, 335-52.

CANCER – skin: See articles CANCER, page 323-25; THE SKIN, page 1769.

CANCER – smear test: See article CANCER, page 321-22.

CANCER – stomach: See articles DIGESTION AND DIGESTIVE DISEASES, page 894; CANCER, pages 326, 335-37.

CANCER – syphilis not related: See article THE VENEREAL DISEASES, page 1952.

CANCER – tar: See article OCCUPATION AND HEALTH, page 1384.

CANCER – testicles: See article CANCER, page 345-47.

CANCER – thyroid: See article ENDOCRINOLOGY, page 682-83.

CANCER – treatment: See articles CANCER, page 322-23; DRUGS AND THEIR USES, page 613-14.

CANCER – uterus: See article CANCER, page 341-44.

CANCER – wens may cause: See article THE SKIN, page 1767.

Cancer

CHARLES S. CAMERON, M.D.

CANCER IN THE PRACTICAL sense is not *a* disease, but rather a large family of diseases having in common the feature of uncontrolled, irregular cell growth, but differing widely in their manifestations, behavior, and response to treatment. This variation in the way cancer expresses itself, especially early in its course, makes its recognition more difficult than is the case with most other diseases. The process of growth is basically one of multiplication of cells—the units of which all living things are composed. Normal, controlled cell division in animal and human life is most active during the period between conception and birth when an entire new organism is being formed. It continues much less rapidly between birth and maturity, after which it slows down to a rate which produces new cells only to replace those which have worn out or have been damaged by disease and injury. For reasons yet unknown, cells occasionally begin to reproduce in the absence of any useful objective; when such purposeless cell division has gone on long enough to produce a mass of cells big enough to be seen or felt, a tumor or new-growth is said to have formed. There are two general kinds of tumor. A *benign* tumor is not very different from the tissue in which it originates and it is clearly separated from the surrounding tissue by a definite capsule. It usually grows slowly and remains in the same area. Such tumors do not endanger life as a rule, they are fairly easily removed and they do not tend to come back. Cancer is a *malignant* tumor. It differs from the tissue of origin in varying degrees. It sends rootlike branches into the normal adjacent

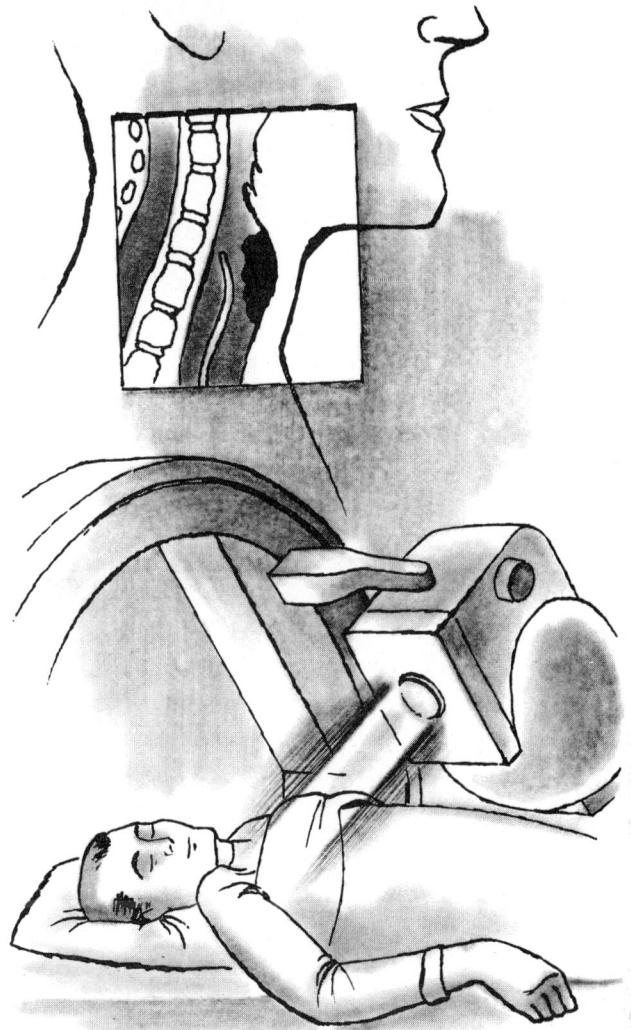

structures, recurs unless every minute bit is removed or destroyed, and, sooner or later, tends to send fragments (metastases) off into distant parts of the body establishing new colonies, identical to the original cancer, which continue to grow. Such aggressive behavior obviously does endanger life. Cancers, in turn, fall into two groups, depending on whether they spring from connective tissue like bone and muscle (sarcoma) or from covering and lining tissue like skin and mucous membrane (carcinoma).

DISTRIBUTION

Cancer and related diseases are found throughout the world of living things. Tumorous growths affect plants, and cancer is familiar to all veterinarians. No race of man is free from it, although statistics from many parts of the world show decided differences in cancer death rates. Where high standards of health result in average long life, cancer is frequent, whereas in countries with poor living standards and high general death rates, people usually do not live long enough to get cancer which is mainly a disease of middle life and beyond. This explains in large measure why cancer has increased so strikingly in our own country in recent years; the proportion of older people in our population is steadily growing, and there are now over three times as many persons past the age of forty-five in the United States as there were in 1900. Control of typhoid fever, meningitis, diphtheria, tuberculosis, pneumonia, and other diseases is leaving little from which to die except heart disease and cancer!

CAUSATIVE FACTORS

While the basic cause of cancer remains unknown, a number of influences seem to favor its development. Among them may be mentioned long-continued exposure to strong sunlight, a factor in skin cancer in the light-complexioned. Cancer of the penis is unknown in males circumcised in infancy although it is seen in others. Cancer of the neck of the womb is commoner among women who have borne children and whose tears have gone unrepaired for years. In certain areas of the world absence of iodine in water and soil gives rise to numerous goiters in which cancer develops more often than it does in normal thyroid glands. Overexposure to the rays of radium and X-ray will result in cancer of the skin, as was the case with many doctors who used these agents before effective methods of protection were known. It is now recognized that heavy, continued cigarette smoking greatly increases the risk of developing cancer of the lung as well as other major diseases. There is no disease about which there are more misconceptions. Cancer is not caused by cooking with gas or by the use of aluminum pots. It is not due to white flour, chemical fertilizers, or hard liquor. In short, it is not a disease of civilization except insofar as civilization permits people to live on into ripe years.

DIAGNOSIS

The more advanced cancer is, the easier it is to identify and, conversely, the smaller or earlier it is, the more difficult diagnosis becomes, although that is when it is most important. The onset of cancer is quiet and gradual, in contrast with many diseases which appear suddenly, dramatically, and demand attention—diseases like appendicitis and pneumonia. Cancer, able to appear anywhere in the body, can manifest itself in a great variety of ways, but the commoner first expressions of the more frequent forms of cancer have been summarized as the Seven Danger Signals of cancer, and they have had an important part in alerting the public to the significance of certain signs and symptoms. They are:

1. Any sore that does not heal (cancer of the skin, lip, or mouth).
2. A lump or thickening in the breast or elsewhere.
3. Unusual bleeding or discharge (cancer of the uterus, rectum, lung, etc.).
4. Any change in a wart or mole.
5. Persistent indigestion (stomach) or difficulty in swallowing (esophagus).
6. Persistent hoarseness (larynx) or cough (lung).
7. Any change in normal bowel habits (rectum or intestine).

Doctors of experience can suspect the presence of many cancers early in their course after analysis of the patient's symptoms and can be reasonably certain of the nature of such tumors as can be seen or felt or visualized by X-ray. Nevertheless, the only completely reliable basis for diagnosing cancer is the biopsy—examination under the microscope of a small portion of the tumor. The procedure of removing a specimen of the tumor for such examination is simple when the tumor is easily accessible as in the skin or lip or neck of the womb (cervix). In other areas such as the rectum, more complicated instruments become necessary, and in such sites as the lung and bladder special skill is required to view and biopsy the lesion. Instruments like these make it possible not only to remove a fragment of the tumor, but to inspect its gross features—an important phase of diagnosis. When cancer arises in the breast, biopsy cannot usually be performed short of a surgical operation, and the same may be said of cancers in most internal organs. The presence of many such internal cancers (stomach, intestine, kidney) is established by X-ray examination, as is the case with cancer of the lung and tumors of the bone. Often X-ray appearance of such tumors offers strong evidence of their nature—strong enough to be used as the basis for treatment.

Recently careful study of individual cells from the surface of cancers has led to the diagnostic method known as the "smear test." The method has proven extremely valuable in determining the nature of tumors of the uterus and lung; it has been somewhat less widely used in studying conditions of the prostate, bladder, kidney, stomach, and large intestine. The smear method does not substitute for the biopsy; it does the scouting—turning up important evidence of cancer, but it remains for the biopsy to establish the final proof of it.

The diagnosis of cancer, then, begins in most cases with the patient himself who correctly interprets a danger signal—trivial though it seems—as a reason to see his doctor. There is no other disease which calls on patients themselves for so large a measure of responsibility for the outcome, because it is the patient himself who must be the first to seek diagnosis at a time when treatment can be successful.

TREATMENT

Effective treatment of cancer is of comparatively recent development. Surgery, as we understand it today, goes back only some seventy-five years, and surgical advances continue to be made as safer anesthesia, better drugs to prevent and combat infection, and wider understanding of nutritional needs make it possible to perform more extensive and hence more curative operations. Indeed, cancer patients are being operated on today, with prospects of cure, who ten years ago would have been classed as altogether hopeless and quite beyond the scope of any kind of treatment. Treatment of cancer by X-rays and radium began as recently as 1895, and much of the technical progress in the field of radiation treatment has grown out of research on atomic energy. X-rays generated by five and ten times the electrical power formerly used are now employed in treatment, and the rays from such machines

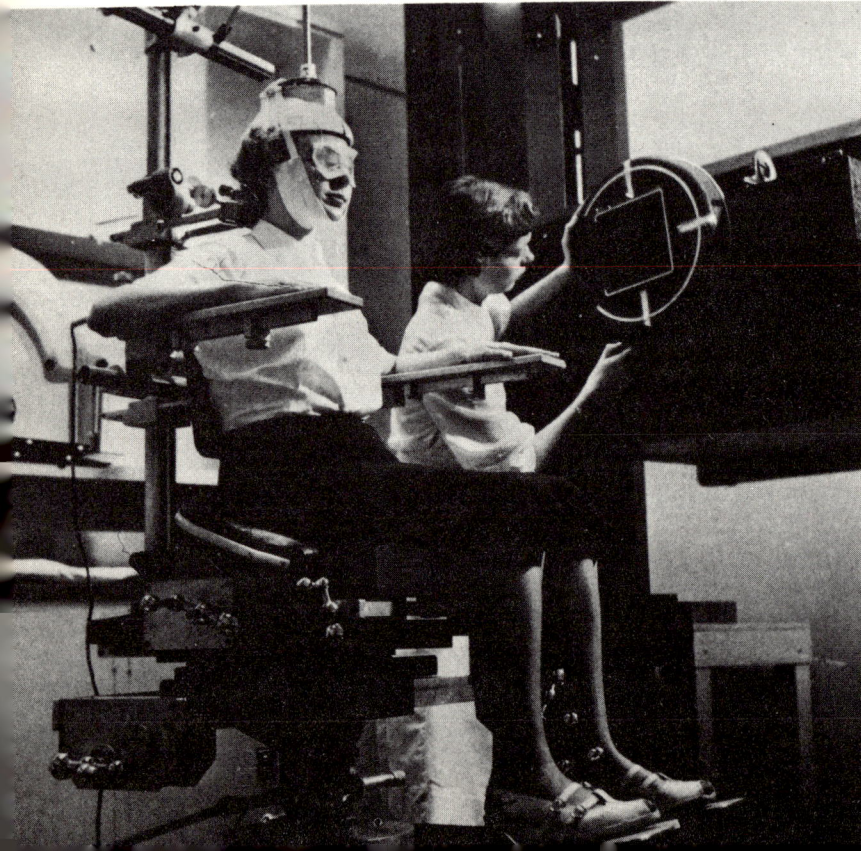

Cancer — Technicians demonstrate rotation radiation, a method that has been used in the treatment of several types of deep-seated cancer. One technician prepares the "eye" of a powerful x-ray beam while another technician "sits in" for the patient. The chair is rotated while the x-ray shoots its cell-destroying rays into the cancer. Surrounding tissues receive only a fraction of radiation because of the rotation while the center of the target gets the maximum effect.

are somewhat more penetrating and therefore more effective in attacking deep-seated cancers. Even stronger are the rays from the atom-smashing betatron. However, it is still too early to say whether such devices will actually cure more cancer.

While surgery, X-rays, and radium (and now radioactive cobalt used like radium) are the only established ways of curing cancer, other methods of treatment have lately come into use. These methods do not cure, but they do make the patient with advanced disease more comfortable and they often pro-long life. Radioactive isotopes provide a means of introducing sources of growth-restraining radiations into the body and, to some degree, selectively into the organ in which cancer is growing (the target). Cancers of a few sex-linked organs, notably the prostate and breast, can be partially controlled in many cases by altering the circulating hormone pattern. This is done by castration (removal of ovaries or testicles) or by giving certain hormones derived from male and female sex glands. Chemical compounds which will restrain the growth of certain kinds of malignant tumors are now used (chemo-therapy) in treating Hodgkin's disease which involves the lymph glands, and leukemia—the overproduction of white blood cells by the blood-forming tissues. As yet no such drug has been found which will do more than relieve symptoms for varying periods. However, even this can be of worth-while benefit, especially in acute leukemia which mostly affects young children and which up to now has been rapidly fatal. Today selected drugs (including ACTH and cortisone) will restore to apparent health up to two thirds of these young patients—always temporarily, but sometimes for over a year.

When cancer is treated is more important than how it is treated. Certainly there is no disease in which the factor of time is of more importance in de-termining the outcome. The differences in the results of treating cancer while it is limited to the organ in which it originated compared to the results once it has begun to spread elsewhere prove beyond doubt, that an early treatment of cancer is of the utmost importance.

QUACKS

The treatment of cancer, by whatever method, is always difficult and exact-ing, calling for the greatest possible experience and skill. Yet there are misguided or unscrupulous persons who belittle the efforts of honest doctors and who claim to have a treatment method far superior to any other. Their methods are usually secret, and the claims made for them are gaudy and assur-ing—such as no self-respecting doctor would dare to make. These cancer quacks sell their diets, pastes, powders, solutions, herbs, and what not to all comers—the hopelessly advanced patients who are grasping at straws and those with early, curable tumors who are trying to avoid the necessary surgical operation. Patients in the latter group lose whatever chance they had of really being cured when they do business with a quack. It must be remembered that it is as unlikely that a person with little understanding of cancer will discover a reliable treatment for it as it would have been for a plumber to have made the atomic bomb.

EARLY SIGNS AND SYMPTOMS

There can be no argument concerning the importance of the early diagnosis of cancer. And since the responsibility of the public in achieving early diagnosis is so great—a responsibility which cannot be delegated to anyone or any agency—all intelligent persons will accept it as their own by familiarizing themselves with the first signs and symptoms of cancer. Although these initial expressions of cancer are indistinguishable from many less serious, even trivial, conditions, a sensible man or woman will not assume that they are unimportant but will take immediate steps to make certain. The following brief description of cancer of various organs is limited to the commoner types and emphasizes those signs and symptoms which appear early and most frequently.

SKIN

Cancer of the skin is commonest of all but fortunately the most curable. It appears usually in the elderly, and those with light or "sandy" complexions seem to be especially prone to it in contrast to persons who tan readily. Negroes rarely have it. The first evidence of a skin cancer is a dry, scaly patch which persists in spite of the usual home remedy—salve of one sort or other. Such lesions are of slow growth, but they do gradually enlarge and involve deeper layers of the skin. As the growth proceeds the scaly surface grows thicker, forming a crust or scab beneath which the area is now found to be raw and moist—the first evidence of ulceration. As the tumor continues to grow its surface becomes fleshy—an open sore, which sometimes bleeds when irritated. It may project above the level of the skin around it or as is more common it may assume crater-like features, the depressed central ulcer being surrounded by an elevated, pearly rim. Skin cancers are apt to develop in warty brown to black lesions which are so common in aging persons, so that changes in such "senile warts" should receive attention. The exposed parts of the body—the face, neck, forearms, and hands—are the favored sites for cancer of the skin. Any sore which does not show signs of healing in a reasonable time, say three weeks, calls for investigation. The usual skin cancer is readily cured by surgical removal, X-ray, or radium. The small ones can even be treated by dessication—thorough destruction with the electric needle.

One kind of cancer usually originating in the skin, although not always, is the pigmented or black cancer called melanoma. Most of these begin in

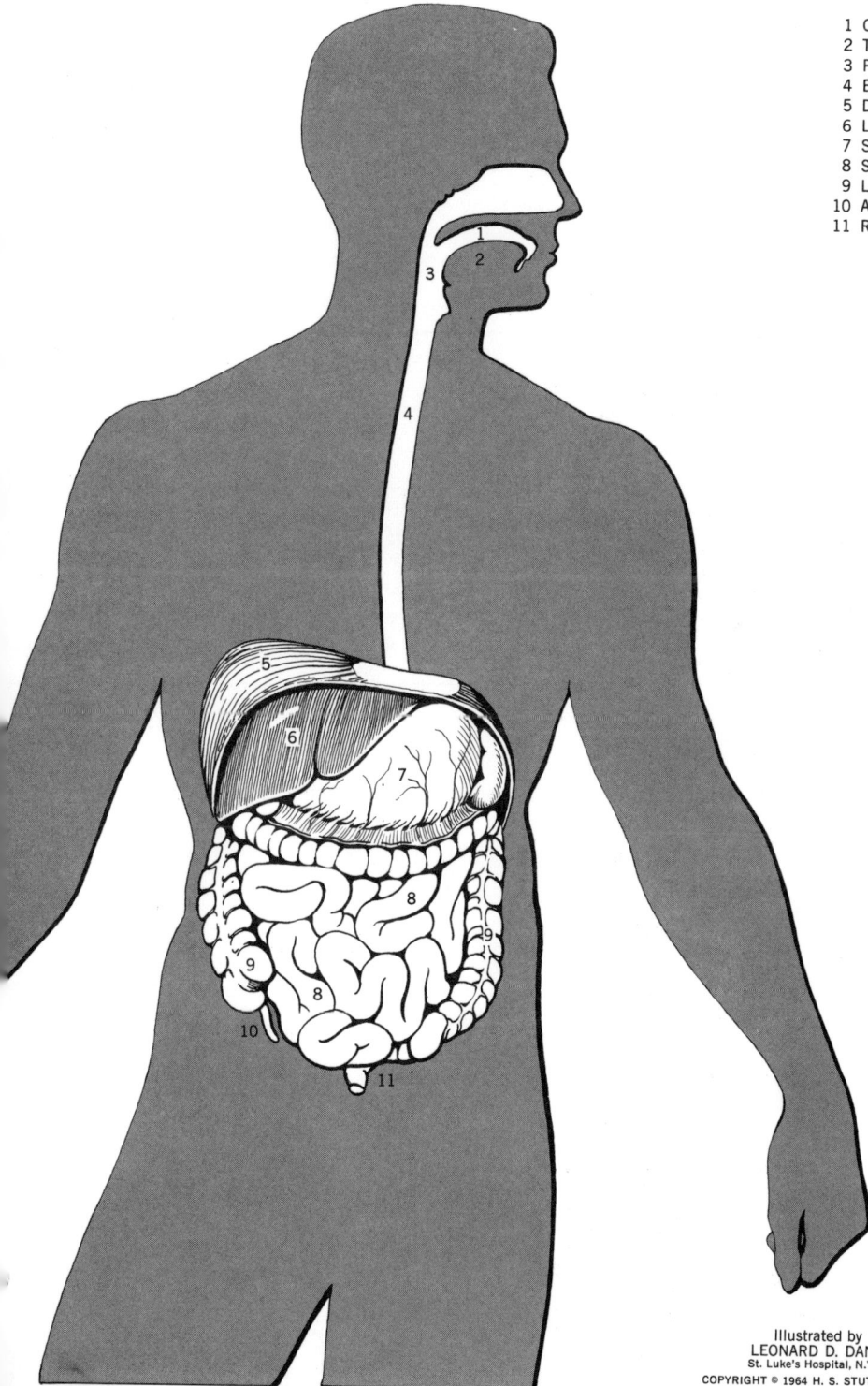

1 ORAL CAVITY
2 TONGUE
3 PHARYNX
4 ESOPHAGUS
5 DIAPHRAGM
6 LIVER
7 STOMACH
8 SMALL INTESTINES
9 LARGE INTESTINES
10 APPENDIX
11 RECTUM

Illustrated by
LEONARD D. DANK
St. Luke's Hospital, N.Y.C.

SALIVARY GLANDS

ESOPHAGUS

LIVER

STOMACH

PANCREAS

SMALL INTESTINE

APPENDIX

LARGE INTESTINE

MOUTH

Digestion begins in the mouth where saliva containing the enzyme ptyalin, starts the breakdown of carbohydrates.

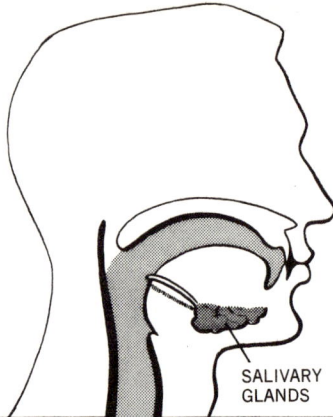

STOMACH

The wall of the stomach contains some 35 million gastric glands. These secrete pepsin and hydrochloric acid which begin the breakdown of proteins.

SMALL INTESTINE

Both the liver and pancreas empty into the small intestine. Bile from liver helps break down fats. Pancreatic secretions are lypase for fats, amylopsin for carbohydrates and trypsin for proteins. The small intestinal walls have millions of glands that secrete similar enzymes.

Absorption of these broken down foods occurs in the lower small intestine. The food passes through the intestinal wall, enters the blood stream and lymph glands for distribution throughout the body.

LARGE INTESTINE

The large intestinal glands secrete mucous to moisten the undigested food which it transports to the anus for elimination.

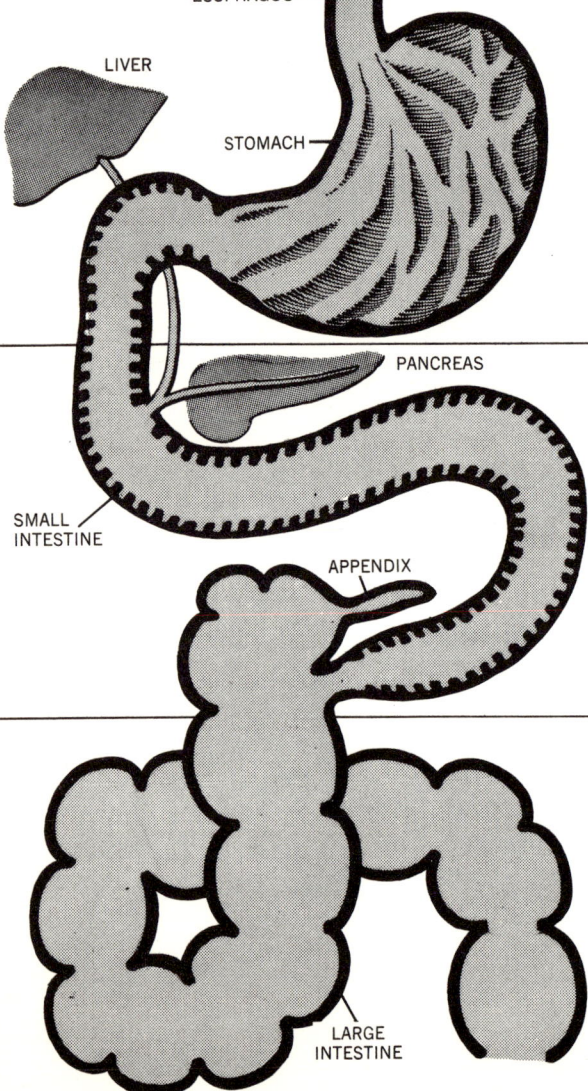

DIGESTIVE SYSTEM III

	CARBOHYDRATES (POTATO-BREAD)	PROTEINS (EGGS-MEATS)	FATS (BUTTER-OILS)
A SALIVARY GLAND 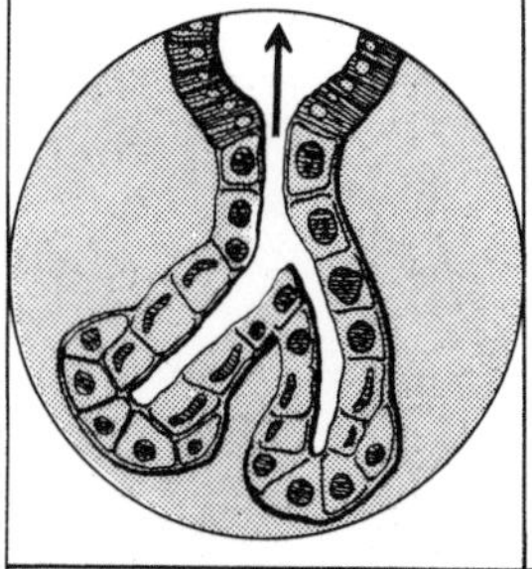	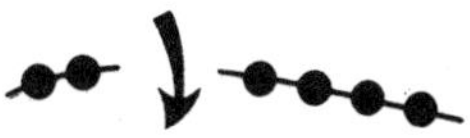 A carbohydrate is a chain of sugars. Ptyalin splits off two-sugar units.	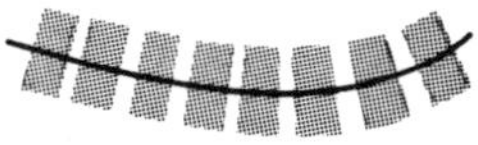 Protein, a chain of amino acids, is unaffected by ptyalin.	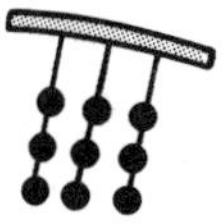 Fat: glycerol plus three fatty acids, is unaffected by ptyalin.
A GASTRIC GLAND 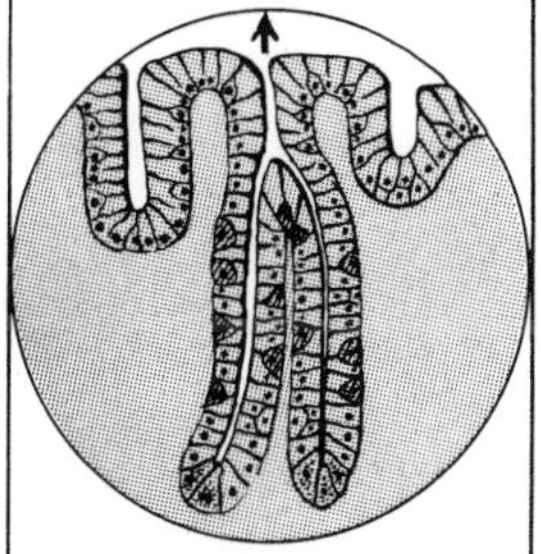	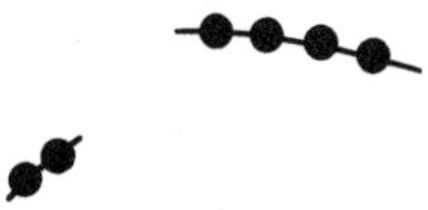 Carbohydrate is unaffected by gastric secretions.	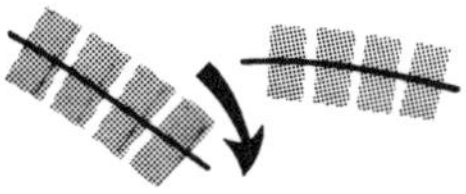 The protein chain is split into smaller units by pepsin and hydrochloric acid.	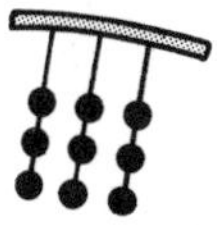 Fat is unaffected by gastric secretions.
SMALL INTESTINAL GLANDS 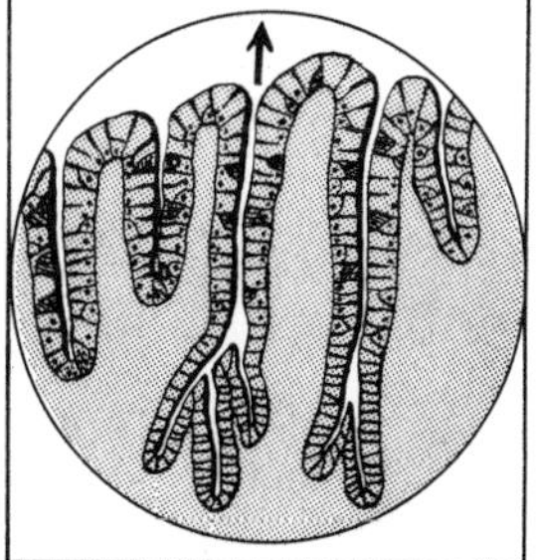	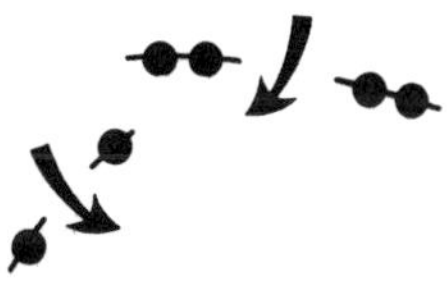 Carbohydrates are broken down to one-sugar units by amylopsin.	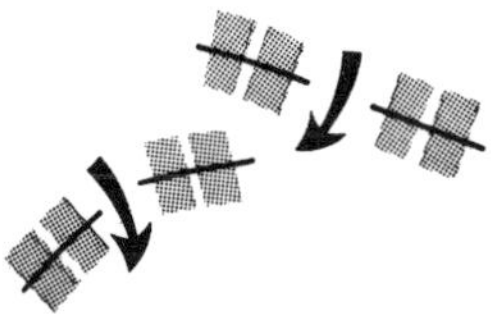 Proteins are broken down into amino acids by trypsin.	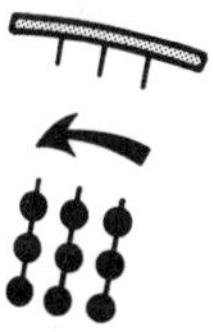 Fat is decomposed into simple units by lipase, aided by the bile.

SMALL INTESTINE

BLOOD VESSEL

LYMPH VESSEL

LARGE INTESTINAL GLANDS

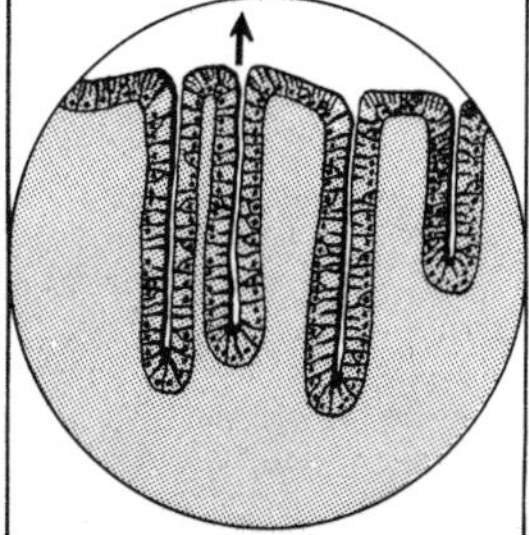

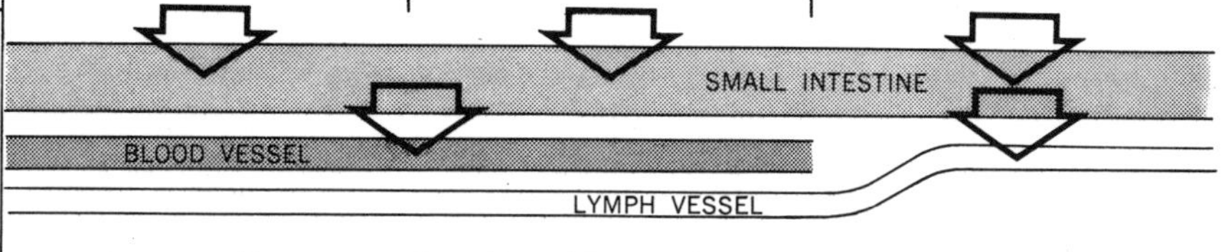

The sugars, amino acids and fats are absorbed by the intestinal wall. Sugars and proteins pass into the blood vessels, while the fat products enter the lymph vessels.

Undigested foods pass into the large intestine, where they are mixed with mucous for lubrication.

DIGESTIVE SYSTEM IV

ESOPHAGUS

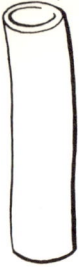

After being masticated by the teeth and mixed with saliva, food is pushed into the pharynx by the tongue. It then enters the esophagus.

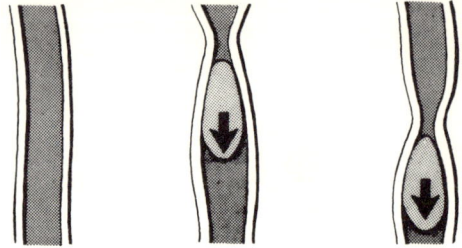

A peristaltic wave moves food through the esophagus.

STOMACH

The muscular stomach walls relax to accommodate the bulk of food.

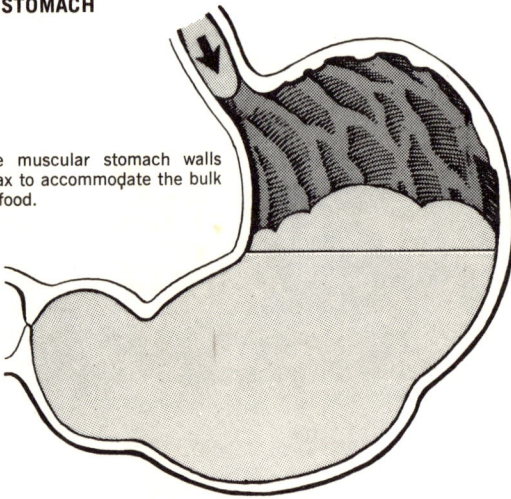

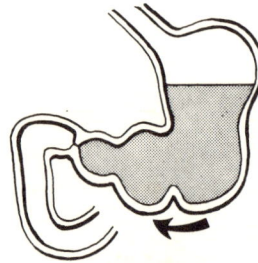

Weak peristaltic waves churn and mix the food with the gastric secretions.

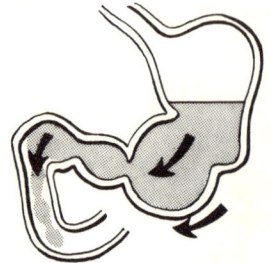

As the peristaltic waves become stronger, the pyloric valve opens, and food enters the small intestine.

SMALL INTESTINE

It takes food 3 to 5 hours to travel the 20 feet of small intestine. The food undergoes 2 types of peristalsis.

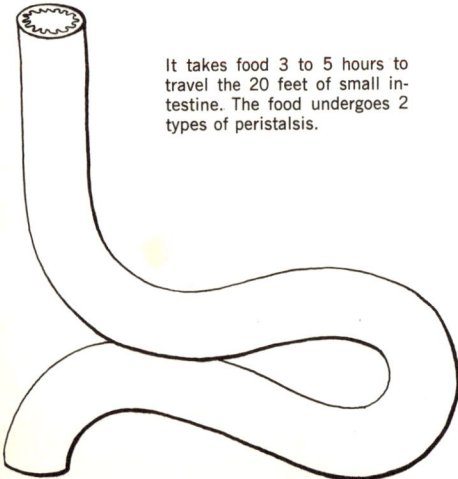

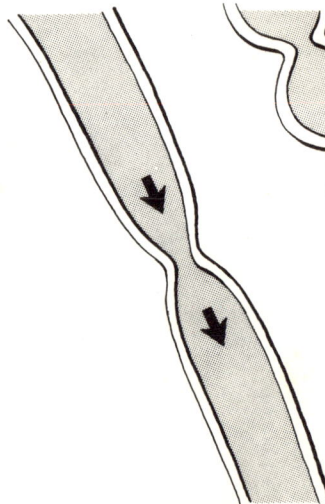

Regular peristaltic movements push the food forward.

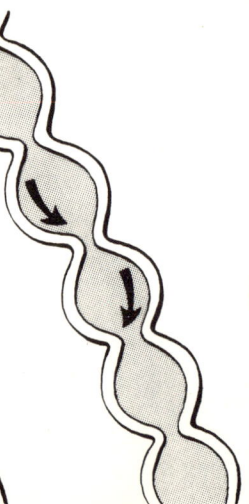

Segmental non-moving contractions churn and mix the food with the intestinal secretions.

THE DIGESTIVE SYSTEM

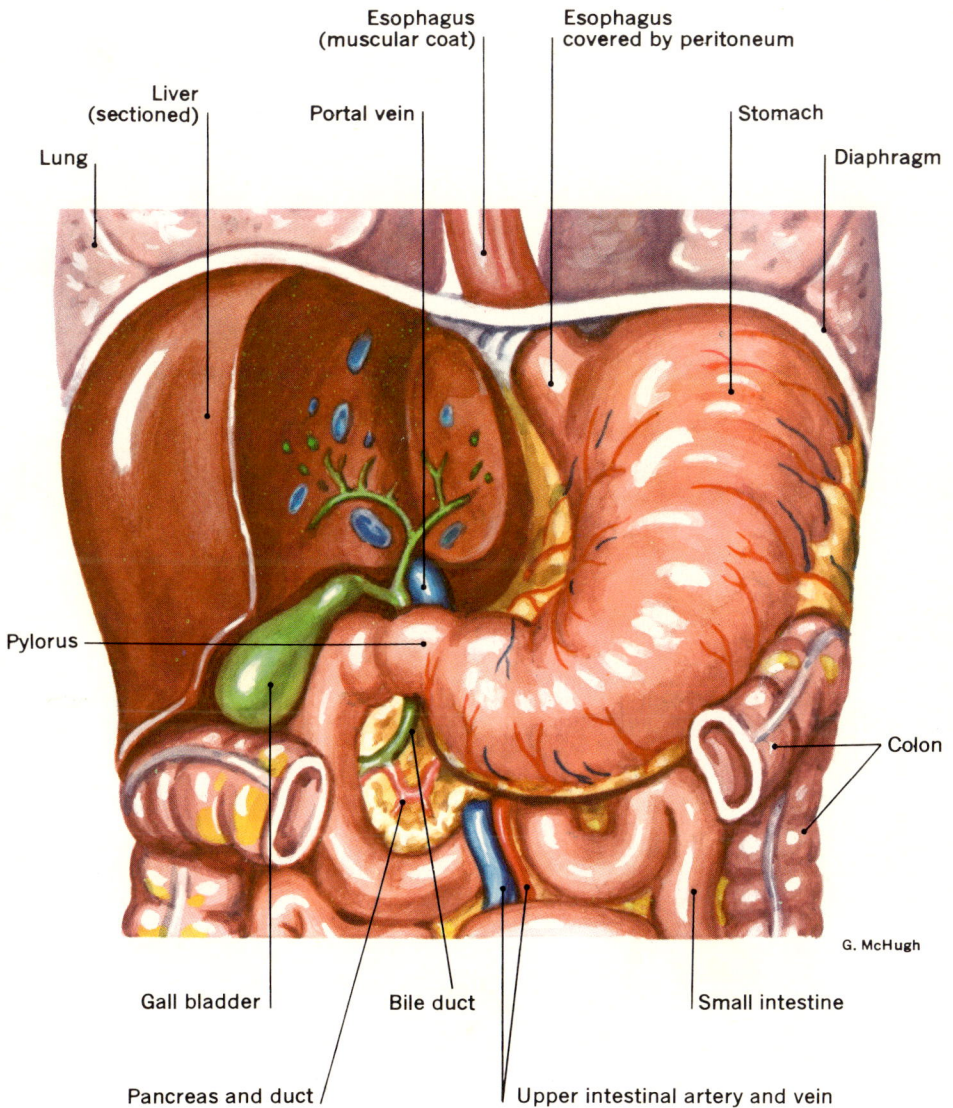

Lung

Liver
(sectioned)

Esophagus
(muscular coat)

Portal vein

Esophagus
covered by peritoneum

Stomach

Diaphragm

Pylorus

Colon

Gall bladder

Bile duct

Small intestine

Pancreas and duct

Upper intestinal artery and vein

G. McHugh

Basically the digestive tract is a long muscular tube, open at both ends, which has specialized parts such as the pouchlike enlargement that forms the stomach. Auxiliary digestive organs are the salivary glands, liver and pancreas which contribute secretions that aid in the breakdown of food. Ducts connect these organs with the digestive tube.

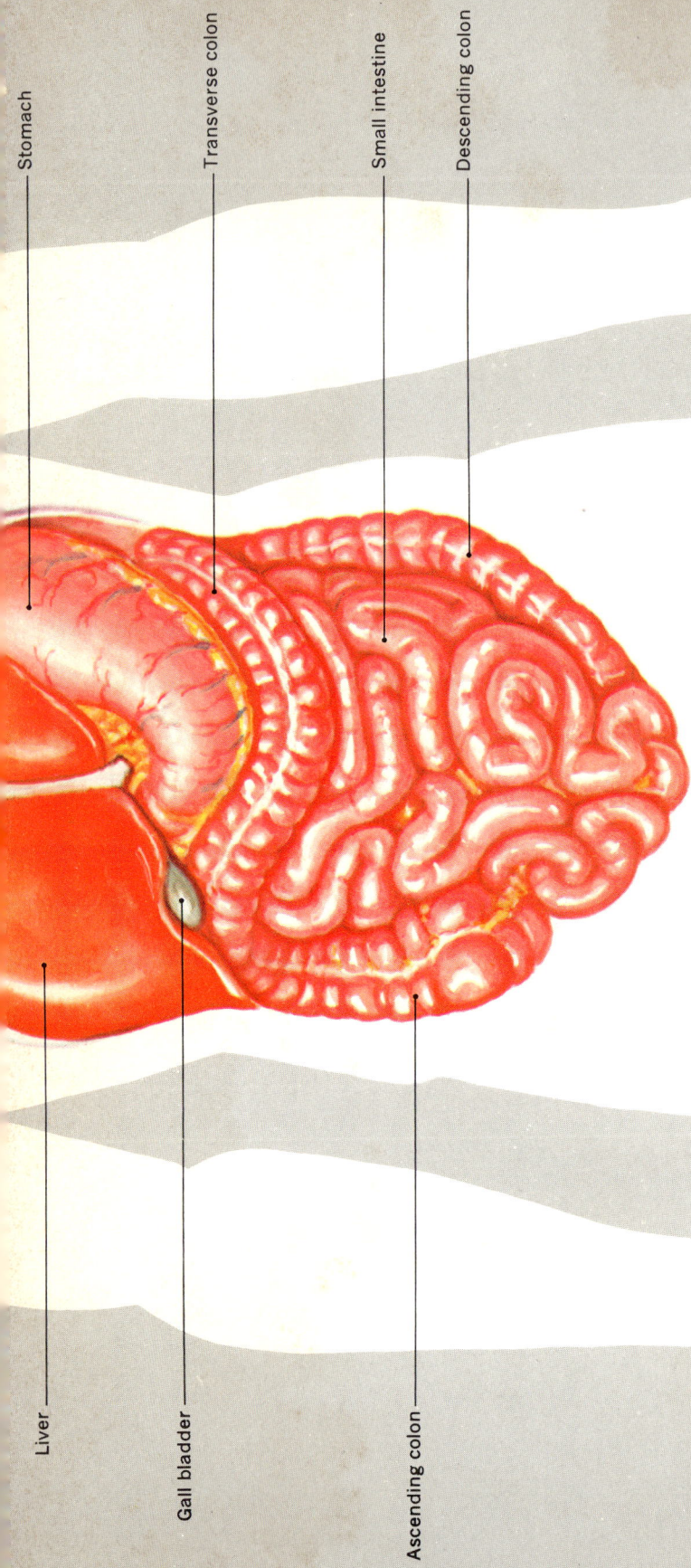

Stomach

Transverse colon

Small intestine

Descending colon

G. McHugh

Liver

Gall bladder

Ascending colon

The Digestive System

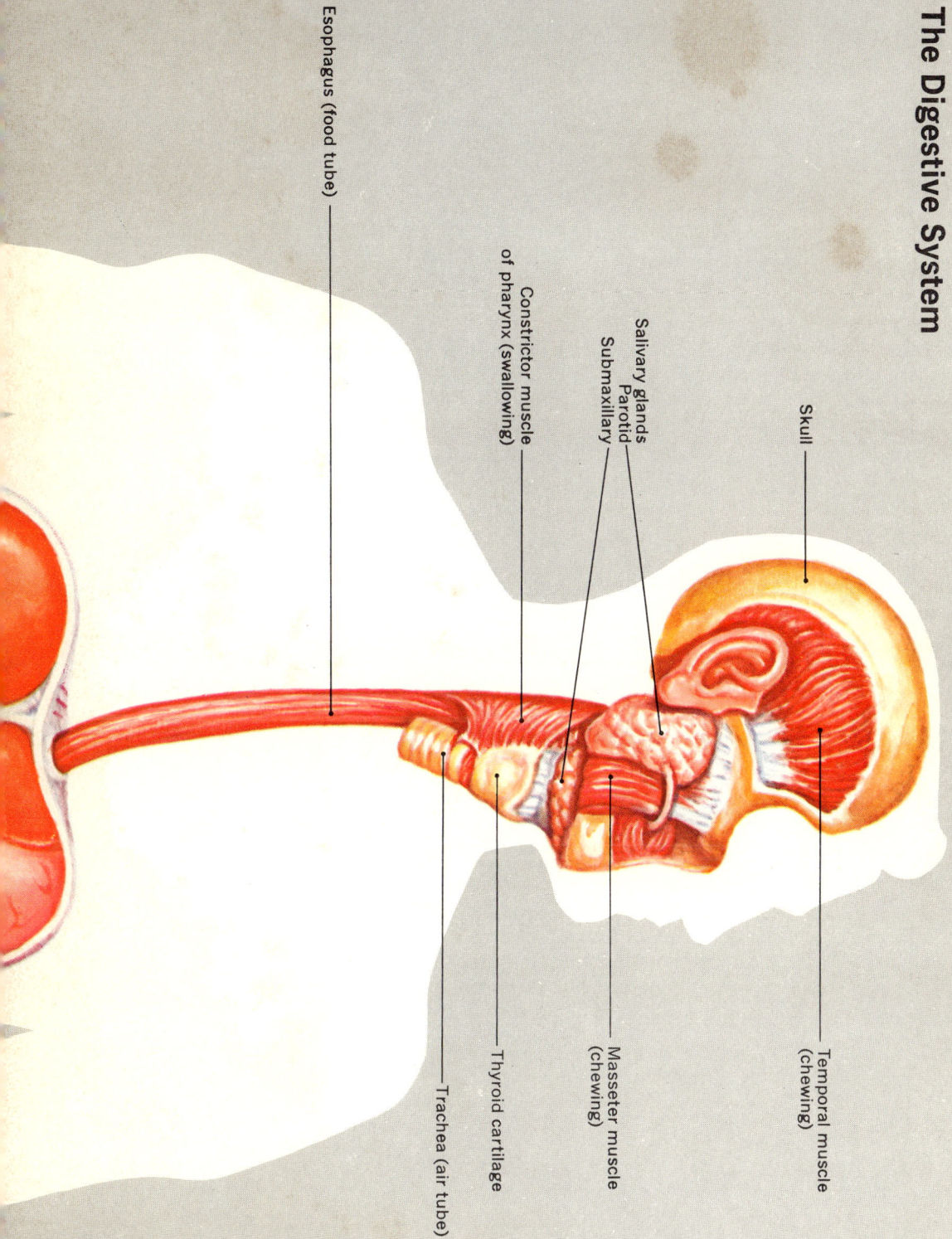

Esophagus (food tube)

Constrictor muscle
of pharynx (swallowing)

Salivary glands
Parotid
Submaxillary

Skull

Trachea (air tube)

Thyroid cartilage

Masseter muscle
(chewing)

Temporal muscle
(chewing)

G. McHugh

Rectum (cut)

Appendix

End of
small intestine

Descending colon

Ascending
colon

Duodenum

Pancreatic duct

Upper mesenteric
artery and vein

Common
bile duct

Pancreas

Gall bladder

Portal vein

Liver

Stomach

Hepatic
veins

Diaphragm

Esophagus

Lung outline

Back View of the Digestive Organs

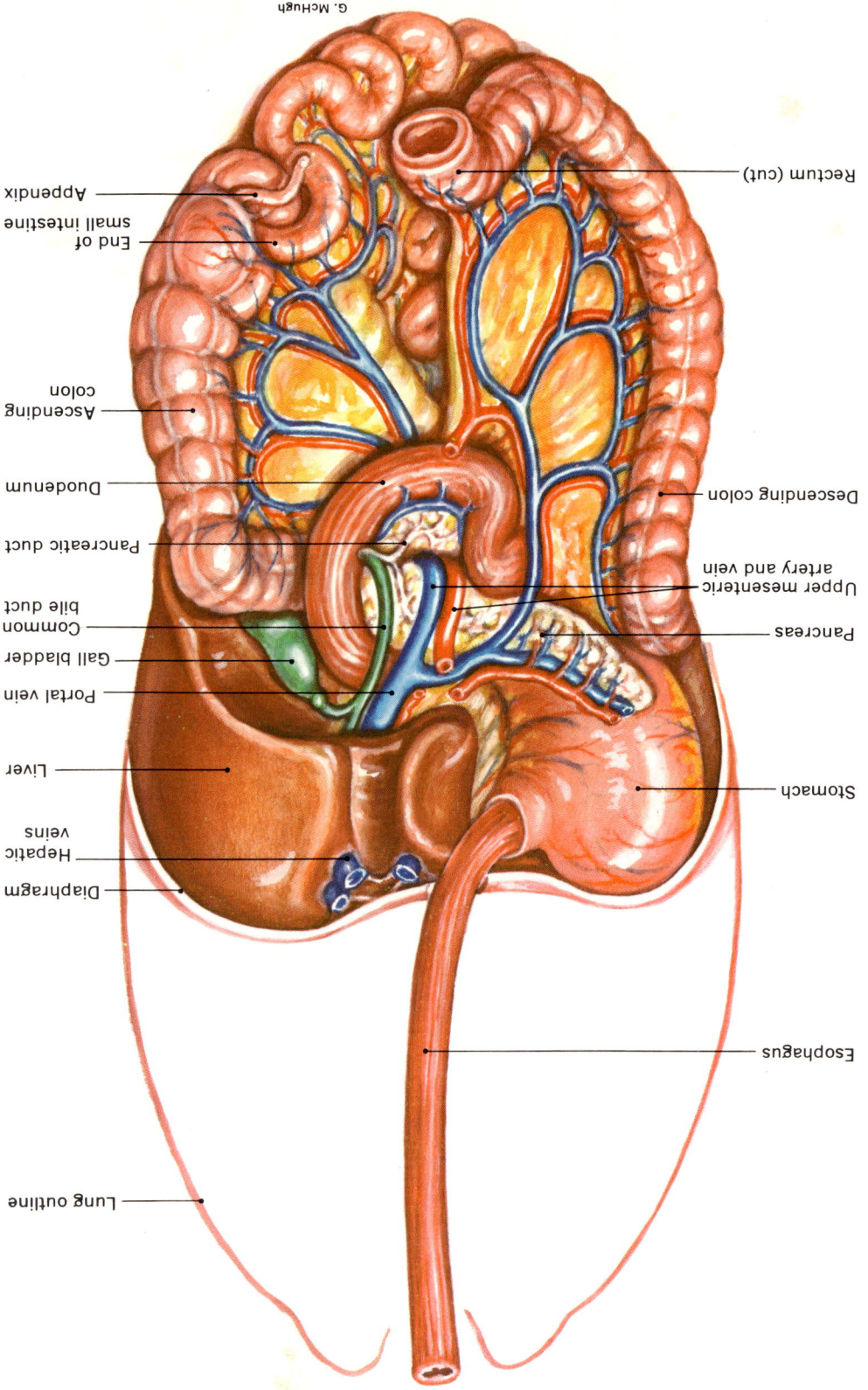

moles, particularly in dark moles, and there is some evidence that injury or repeated irritation of such moles may play a part in converting them to cancer. Melanoma begins most often as an enlargement of a pre-existing mole, and at the same time its color deepens; the lesion becomes raised, and ulceration with slight bleeding is apt to appear. Removal of pigmented lesions showing signs of such activity is immediately imperative. They should never be cauterized with the electric needle. Melanoma is a relatively rare tumor—a fact of much comfort, since the average person has twenty-one moles! Nevertheless, it is a wise health practice to have moles removed which are located where they are apt to be irritated.

Circumstances favoring the development of cancer of the skin are (1) fair complexion, with skin which sunburns repeatedly rather than tanning; (2) prolonged exposure to strong sunlight, and (3) overexposure to hot, dry wind with its drying effect on normal skin oils. Therefore, the only established preventive measure is avoidance of repeated and long-continued exposure to these influences, especially by those with fair skins. The skin cancers which result from exposure to arsenic, lubricating oils, and other substances involved in specific occupations are of little importance to the average person.

LIP AND MOUTH

The features of skin cancer previously described are often the same for cancer of the lip, which is nearly always on the lower lip. A scaly area appearing whitish in contrast to the vermilion lip surface, and which shows no tendency to heal but rather to enlarge slowly, suggests the possibility of cancer. The crust may grow thicker or may give way to a frank ulcer of varying depth, usually surrounded by a thickened elevated rim. Sometimes, however, as the lesion progresses the growth of cells piles up, layer upon layer, so that a mass of tissue protrudes well above the surface. The latter type is prone to have an irregular, pebbly or granular surface and has therefore been compared to a cauliflower. Cancer of the lip quite often develops in and is preceded by a condition of the membrane of the lip known as leukoplakia, which literally means white plaque. Leukoplakia has the appearance of a thin, white film or sometimes it resembles a bit of wet white tissue paper. It is not cancer—being merely a thickening of the layers of the lip's covering —but in certain cases it becomes cancerous. Like cancer of the skin, lip cancer is treated by surgical removal or by X-rays or radium. Because it is a frequent forerunner of cancer, leukoplakia should also be treated promptly. Excessive exposure to strong sunlight is the chief causative factor in cancer of the lip, and, therefore, as in the case of the skin, protection of the lip from its direct rays is the sole accepted preventive.

Cancer of the mouth may involve the tongue, gum, floor of the mouth, inner surface of the cheek, or the palate (roof of the mouth). It may take the form of (1) an ulcer or "sore," (2) a raised, irregular, warty area, or (3) a lump or thickening. Such changes are frequently felt first by the tongue and should invite inspection in a mirror. Of course almost everyone has experienced sores in the mouth which after a few days or so disappear of themselves. The clue to the importance of any lesion in the mouth is its persistence beyond two weeks, and any such sore or lump which does not show a tendency to heal within that time should be seen without further delay by a doctor or dentist. Irregularities of the mucous surface of the mouth are sometimes caused by sharp, jagged teeth, especially broken teeth, or by poorly fitting bridges or plates. Although the cause of such lesions may appear clear to the patient, they should not be disregarded, and all such sources of irritation should be corrected. Leukoplakia occurs in the mouth, as on the lip, and it occurs more often in the mouths of heavy smokers. In fact, such white areas used to be called "smoker's patch." Since leukoplakia is so often precancerous, it must be taken seriously and eliminated. Sometimes it is enough to stop smoking, and in other cases vitamin therapy is indicated. But usually surgical treatment by excision or cauterization is necessary.

The factors widely regarded as tending to cause cancer of the mouth are (1) abuse of tobacco, (2) poor mouth hygiene, (3) sharp teeth or improperly fitting dentures, and (4) habitual ingestion of very hot food and liquid. These causes do not have as much proof as they ought to have in order to condemn them fairly, but their correction is so simple as to invite precaution even though proof of their rôle is lacking. Therefore, to reduce the likelihood of mouth cancer, if you must smoke keep it in moderation; keep your mouth clean by following your dentist's advice to brush the teeth twice daily; do not permit broken teeth or chafing dental appliances to go uncorrected; avoid insulting your mouth with food and drink which is too hot.

LARYNX

The cancers discussed so far can be seen and not heard, but the opposite is true for cancer of the voice box. It is not visible (to the patient), it cannot be felt with the tongue or finger, but it does give a sign of its presence which can be heard. That sign is hoarseness. Fortunately, in most cases this warning note is sounded early in the development of the growth. Hoarseness which develops without reasonable cause demands prompt examination of the larynx. Yet delay is the general rule; in fact, the average patient with cancer of the larynx waits three and a half months after hoarseness develops before consulting a doctor. To be sure, hoarseness is a common accompaniment of colds, and it is not unusual for it to hang on for a short time afterward. But any hoarseness—no matter from what apparent cause—which lasts for three weeks is cause for careful medical examination. The high rate of curability of early larynx cancer (nine out of ten cases confined to one chord are cured) makes early diagnosis of unquestioned lifesaving value. There are no generally accepted causes of this form of cancer, although it is claimed by some that it occurs somewhat more frequently among heavy smokers. Again, moderation in smoking appears to be the only available prophylaxis.

ESOPHAGUS

Cancer of the esophagus or gullet is fairly uncommon. The structure of the organ is such that diagnosis early in the disease is achieved all too rarely, and so it is among the more fatal forms of cancer. The chief symptom is difficulty in swallowing. At first this is slight, and food seems to hesitate for a moment on the way down, after which it progresses to the stomach. This sensation that food is sticking occurs in the beginning with bulky, dry foods such as bread and certain meats. Later the passage of all solid foods becomes delayed and eventually even liquids. Spasm of the irritated esophagus and actual obstruction by tumor are responsible for these signs. Treatment is by surgical removal in favorable cases and by deep X-ray treatment when the growth is more advanced. Recently X-rays generated at high voltage and the high energy particles emanating from the betatron have shown somewhat greater restraint of cancer of the esophagus and other deep-lying tumors, but it does not yet appear that actual cures can be obtained with them. There are no known causes of this variety of cancer which operate generally, although the somewhat higher than average rate in northern Scandinavian countries has been attributed to a diet deficient in vitamin B. This complex of vitamins appears necessary to maintain mucous membranes in a healthy condition, and when it is restricted or absent from the diet generative changes (including leukoplakia) may occur in these tissues.

STOMACH

Cancer of the stomach is, or was until recently, responsible for more deaths than any other form of cancer, one in every eight cancer deaths being charged to it. Two facts account for this high mortality—its frequency and the relatively small number of cases operated on in time to permit removal of all the disease. The delay before the diagnosis is made is appalling. Of all patients who develop cancer of the stomach, fewer than half are found to be suitable for operation—they are clearly too late. Of those who are operated on, fewer than half are found to have disease which can be removed. These are the patients of whom it is said, "They opened him and closed him right away." Again, too late. Of the remaining few who have a chance and on whom a complete operation can be done, a few more will die before leaving the hospital. Finally a small group who could be operated on, whose tumors could be removed, and who survived the surgical procedure, are left. But they are not yet all cured, for within five years well over half of them will succumb to recurring cancer—to the hidden remnants of disease which eluded removal.

All this adds up to the forlorn fact that of all patients who get cancer of the stomach, not more than 5 or 6 per cent are living free of the disease five years later. But this gloomy picture is not without its hopeful aspect, for much of the high mortality is due to the fact that these cancers are not usually diagnosed until late in their course, and some of this delay, perhaps a very important—even critical—part of it, should be susceptible of substantial reduction. The silent interval of cancer of the stomach—the period from its actual beginning to the appearance of signs and symptoms—may be as long as twenty months. Barring the discovery of a reliable, simple, and cheap diagnostic test, it does not seem likely that this portion of the delay period can be influenced. But after the development of digestive complaints, the average patient with cancer of the stomach waits another eight months before deciding to consult a doctor. This eight months, over which the patient and the patient alone has control, must be relied on for reducing the fateful interval between onset and treatment.

The bright side of the coin is that when cancer of the stomach is treated while the disease involves the stomach only (before lymph node spread has occurred), five-year cures in over 50 per cent are to be expected, and one large clinic has recently reported 64 per cent of such patients alive and well five years after operation. This is a heartening figure, especially when it is compared to the five-year results among the patients whose primary cancers were removed but where lymph node spread was present—only 12 per cent of whom lived beyond the five-year mark, and among the entire stomach cancer group, of which not more than one in twenty are living and well five years after they are stricken.

The opportunity to relieve this situation lies in the greatest possible reduction of the delay interval following the onset of stomach symptoms. Undoubtedly many lives could be saved if the average waiting time were to be cut to three or four weeks instead of the present seven or eight months. It is not easy to spot the symptoms of early cancer of the stomach because most of us have some mild stomach complaints from time to time and have come to accept them as the consequences of "something that didn't agree with me," or too much drinking, too much smoking, or overwork and what not. And most times we have been right. One has only to listen to the radio for a few hours or read a single magazine or newspaper to realize that "acid indigestion," "sour stomach," "heartburn," and "dyspepsia" must be widespread indeed to call for such numerous remedies as are advertised so intensively. So they are! The danger lies right here: the symptoms of simple indigestion or dyspepsia are no different from the early symptoms of cancer of the stomach. Perhaps the single term most expressive of the complaints of patients with stomach cancer is indigestion. True, this covers a multitude of conditions, and it is not a precise word—meaning different things to different people. On the other hand, its general coverage makes it useful to the public in describing the varied and subtle details of symptoms which may arise in the abdomen. "Indigestion," then, may be another way of describing (1) a vague sense of unease referable to the stomach, (2) a feeling of fullness or bloating, (3) mild nausea, (4) heartburn, (5) lessening of the normal healthy appetite, which often appears first as quick satiation—the feeling that one has eaten all he can after a few mouthfuls of food, (6) eructation of food, (7) excessive belching, and (8) pain. At the onset these symptoms are vague and they may be inconstant, coming and going with or without the usual medicine-cabinet remedies. How long then can one safely temporize? If a man or woman over forty years of age who has not had previous more or less chronic stomach trouble develops indigestion which lasts for two weeks, the possibility of serious organic disease is to be thought of, and even though such complaints will prove in most cases to have been due to something other than cancer, the wise man or woman will let the doctor determine the cause of the trouble.

There is another expression of cancer of the stomach which occurs often enough to be worth remembering. Shortness of breath from mild exertion, and fatigue from activity which formerly caused no tiring may be the first signs of this disease. They result from anemia which follows repeated small amounts of bleeding from the ulcerated portion of the stomach, and sometimes the quantity of blood lost is sufficient to produce obvious paleness. With older people who have had ulcers and "nervous stomachs" for years, the recognition of indigestion due to cancer is confused by the merging of their old complaints with the new. Of course, if chronic stomach symptoms change their character, become more intense or more frequent, suspicion should be aroused, but such changes are apt to be so gradual that a clear transition is rarely recognized.

Perhaps the best course for those past middle life with chronic stomach trouble and without it is to give the doctor a chance twice a year to re-evaluate the status of the digestive system. Let him be the judge of what tests if any need to be done. Let him share with you the responsibility of finding cancer early—which is another way of saying let him help you to live long and stay well.

INTESTINES

Cancer occurs less often in the small intestine than in the large, and when it affects the small bowel, its symptoms or warning signs are less definite and hence more difficult to interpret than is the case with tumors in the colon (large intestine). For this reason cancer of the small intestine has a less favorable outcome than that of the colon.

One of the earlier symptoms common to both is increased intestinal gas, that is, more than is usual, considering individual variations. Gas may be formed in such quantities as to cause discomfort varying from mild uneasiness to frank cramps. The content of the small bowel is liquid, so tumors here do not produce the signs of obstruction until they have almost closed off the intestinal passage. As greater obstruction is caused by the growing tumor, the symptoms of crampy pain often relieved by the passage of gas, and a change of bowel habits expressed by increasing constipation or diarrhea, become more insistent. Surgical removal of the tumor-bearing portion of the intestine is the one treatment, and when the growth is confined to the bowel the results are good.

The content of the large intestine is solid as compared to that of the small, and it becomes progressively more solid as it passes from the cecum at the beginning of the colon through the large bowel to the rectum. The solider the fecal mass is, the less obstruction is required to interfere with it and thereby produce symptoms. Therefore, as a general rule, the closer to the rectum a tumor of the colon is, the earlier symptoms will be produced and, theoretically at least, the more favorable the prospect for treatment in time. Cancers of the large intestine are associated usually with unusual quantities of gas, with varying degrees of abdominal discomfort or outright pain—usually not steady but appearing at first quite irregularly, later becoming more frequent and assuming the rhythm of cramps. This variety of cancer is apt to ulcerate early so that bleeding occurs in small amounts. This bleeding may be too slight to appear as blood in the stool (although chemical tests will reveal it) yet, continued week in and week out, it is often enough to cause a significant degree of anemia. The patient may look pale in the more severe cases; he may complain of fatigue, shortness of breath, or weakness; and in each case the blood count will confirm the existence of anemia. So consistently is anemia a feature of cancer of the colon that every patient having anemia without obvious cause should have careful X-ray studies of the intestine. When bleeding is sufficient to appear in the stool, the location of the tumor will determine how it appears. If the tumor is in the first portion of the colon —the part farthest from the rectum—the blood will be dark and will have become thoroughly mixed with the feces so that the stool will appear dark. The nearer the tumor is to the rectum or anus, the brighter the blood will be, and the more it will be separated from the stool itself, so that bleeding from cancer of the rectum located within six or eight inches of the anal opening will present as frank blood as seen in the toilet or on the tissue. A change in the bowel habits is apt to occur. Constipation, not previously troublesome, may develop; yet because of the irritation of the tumor and the production of larger quantities of mucus, diarrhea is also common; and often the two alternate.

Summarizing, the important early signs of cancer of the rectum and large intestine are (1) bleeding, seen in the stool or causing anemia or both, (2) a persistent change in the usual bowel habits—diarrhea or constipation or both, and (3) increased intestinal gas causing varying degrees of abdominal discomfort.

Surgical removal of the segment of the intestine involved by the cancer gives excellent results when the tumor is discovered and treated while it is confined to the bowel wall. Indeed, cures in 75 per cent of patients with cancer of the rectum treated while the disease was limited to the mucous lining have been reported.

With a single exception, causes of cancer of the rectum and large intestine have not been recognized. This exception is a precancerous condition known as polyposis, and it consists of the presence of small benign tumors called polyps which arise in and hang from the lining of the intestine or rectum. They may be solitary, but more often there are more than one, and occasionally there are many scattered along the length of the large bowel. Although not cancer, these polyps tend to become malignant as time goes on, and for this reason their removal or destruction is of great importance. Intestinal polyps tend to run in families; therefore it is a wise precaution for anyone who has had a parent or grandparent affected by cancer of the rectum or colon to seek a careful examination of his lower intestinal tract, including studies by X-ray.

BREAST

This is the cancer most feared by women, and for good reason, as it is the commonest major form of cancer among them. It is most likely to occur after the age of forty-five or fifty, although, as cancers go, it is not rare in the thirties. The first evidence of breast cancer is a lump in the breast, and this lump is usually painless. It may be present in any part of the breast, but the upper outer quarter is favored. As the mass of cancer grows larger, other signs appear. There may appear a suggestion of flattening of the normal convexity of the breast outline which later comes to look like obvious dimpling. The nipple may sink downward or "retract," and in time come to lie entirely beneath the adjacent skin level. Or, as the result of the pull exerted on the nipple by the tumor, the nipple may change its axis by tilting in the direction of the tumor. Later a portion of the skin covering the breast or much of it may grow tense, with the pores becoming prominent so that it resembles the skin of an orange. As the tumor grows to occupy more space, the breast may become larger, as would seem natural, but just as often it appears to shrivel, a paradox caused by the replacement of normally elastic tissue by the dense, hard tissue of cancer. Bleeding or other discharge from the nipple occurs when cancer develops in the larger ducts of the breast close to the nipple, but such abnormal nipple discharge is more often due to a benign tumor in a duct. But there is no way to know which it is—benign or malignant—short of surgical exploration, which is why operation is urged in all instances of bleeding nipple. Of course, benign tumors of the breast, which are very frequent, also present themselves as lumps so that the mere fact of a breast mass does not always mean cancer, and in women under fifty it usually does not. Again, examination by an experienced doctor will suggest the nature of the mass as a rule; but doctors with the greatest experience with breast tumors are the most ardent advocates of surgical removal of all true tumors arising therein, for microscopic examination is after all the most dependable and accurate of all diagnostic methods.

When the complete operation of removal is performed at a time when cancer is confined to the breast, the likelihood of cure is 80 to 90 per cent. When cancer has spread to the lymph glands in the armpit, as it is apt to do, there is still a worthwhile chance for cure, but it has dropped to 30 per cent or so. The administration of deep X-rays following surgery for breast cancer is widely employed in select cases.

The causes of breast cancer are unknown. A number of observers have recorded a lower rate of breast cancer among women who have borne children than those who have not, and a lower rate among women who have breast-fed their children than among those who have not. If any conclusion at all is justified on the basis of this evidence, it would be that the use of the breasts in fulfilment of their essential purpose is better than interruption of their normal function. The answer to the problem of breast cancer is to find and treat it before it has metastasized. This is not always possible, because some tumors spread to other parts of the body before they have grown large enough to be discovered. But the principle of "the earlier, the better" should nevertheless guide our approach to all cancer control, including the control of cancer of the breast.

Consider the fact that the average woman with this disease first consults a doctor at a time when the tumor measures roughly two inches across—about the size of a golf ball. This is a good-sized mass, and the question immediately arises, "Why do they wait so long?" The fact is that many of these women do not wait; rather, their oft-repeated story is, "I found this lump a few nights ago," and they usually add, "while I was taking a bath." In other words, they found the lump *accidentally*. Recently a number of doctors have wondered whether such women could not have found a lump many months before it grew to the size of a golf ball—when it would have been smaller, to be sure—if they had taken the trouble to deliberately feel for one. The answer is clearly yes. Experience has shown women can feel breast tumors as small as half an inch in diameter—indeed, can discover lumps so small that the doctor himself has difficulty identifying them. Six to twelve months are required for a breast cancer to grow from a size which can just be found to the size usually encountered at the time of surgery. Precious, wasted months—months of delay which could have been avoided! This delay can be avoided by any woman intelligent enough to adopt the practice of regularly methodically examining her own breasts once a month. The day following the end of each menstrual period should be checked as the proper time to perform the examination, but as the danger of breast cancer does not cease with the change of life, the practice should be continued on a monthly basis throughout life. An instructive film illustrating the proper technique of self-examination has been produced by the American Cancer Society and the National Cancer Institute and shown widely to audiences of women throughout the country. The essential steps in the examination, which need take no more than five minutes.

Any sensible woman, examining her own breasts regularly, will become thoroughly familiar with their structural features, and she can be relied on to recognize even very slight departures from this normal structure. Any such development must be brought to her doctor's attention at once. As has been said, not all breast cancers can be cured—even with early treatment—but it is possible that the general recognition of them while they are still very small would double the number of cures now being achieved. Everyone agrees to the value of brushing the teeth daily—and everyone does it. Yet judged by the standard of its lifesaving potential, monthly self-examination of the breasts is vastly more important.

UTERUS

Cancer of the womb is only slightly less frequent than cancer of the breast, and each year some 45,000 women develop it. It occurs about eight times more often in the cervix or neck of the womb than it does in the cavity or body of the uterus. In either case its cardinal warning sign is irregular bleeding from the vagina. When such abnormal bleeding appears during the active menstrual life, it may take the form of bleeding between the regular menstruations, or it may present as excessively heavy or prolonged monthly flow. Such irregularities are too often attributed to some minor cause—to a "cold" or irritation or to the beginning of the "change." When vaginal bleeding occurs after the change of life, its wholly unexpected appearance leaves little of excuse for failing to interpret it as an event calling for prompt investigation, for cancer is the most important, probably the most frequent, cause of bleeding at such a time. And yet even here mistakes are made; too many women are prone to interpret the unexpected flow as a "return of the monthly," and even to welcome it as an indication that they are not as old as they thought they were. It is during the menopause when bleeding is not according to schedule that the greatest confusion arises, and it may be difficult indeed to distinguish correctly the abnormal irregularity of bleeding due to a tumor from the normal irregularity attributable to the change of life.

While irregular bleeding is the foremost warning sign of uterine cancer, such bleeding need not consist of dark or bright red blood, though it often does. A vaginal discharge which develops in a woman of any age may be present in cancer, especially of the body of the womb, so that the cause of all discharges should be carefully sought. Vaginal discharge, while not uncommon and often due to benign conditions, is nevertheless always abnormal, and its cause should be determined and corrected. But when cancer is present in the uterus, the discharge is tinged with blood as a rule, and its color may vary from the faintest pink to the deep red of frank blood. Fortunately, women have the advantage of a method of protection against illness and death from cancer of the womb; the core of the control of this widespread disease lies in persuading *all* women to accept this protection. It consists of a thorough pelvic examination performed twice a year, even though there are no signs or complaints referable to the pelvis. It is not necessary for women to wait for abnormal bleeding to mark the presence of cancer—because such cancers can be found by meticulous search before they give rise to any signs whatever. In fact, it is now possible to identify cancer of the cervix before it can be seen by the eye of the examining doctor.

A pelvic examination is not difficult for the physician or unpleasant for the patient and takes but a few minutes to carry out. In the course of it the doctor will inspect all of the generative organs which can be seen—the vulva, the vaginal tube, and, most important, the cervix, that portion of the uterus which projects into the upper vagina. He will then examine the cervix with his fingers, and with his hands the pelvic organs which cannot be viewed— the body of the uterus, the ovaries, the tubes, and the adjacent supporting structures. He will possibly include a vaginal smear in his survey—a relatively new development which holds much promise for earlier diagnosis of malignant tumors of the uterus. By withdrawing a little secretion from the upper vagina and from the opening of the cervix and by staining the cells with special dyes, the nature of the cells present in the smear can be determined with a high degree of accuracy. Specifically, when cancer is present in the cervix, cancer cells can usually be seen in the smear; the reliability of the smear in cancer of the body of the uterus is slightly less than in cervix cancer. Of course, there is little difficulty in spotting cancer of the cervix when it is large enough to be seen and felt—that is, when it has been present long enough to be unmistakable. But when this stage is reached the outlook is often less favorable. The exciting feature of the smear method is that it can reveal or strongly suggest the presence of cancers so small that they cannot readily be seen or felt; and of course such cancers are early and highly curable. Smears are also of great value in identifying cancer in a cervix which is already so distorted by co-existing benign disease—tears, infection, and inflammation—that the malignant process is obscured.

The woman who is wise enough to play it safe, then, will do more than be alert for the danger signal of cancer of the uterus—abnormal bleeding or discharge; she will act before such signals have a chance to appear, by insisting upon a careful examination of her pelvis twice a year—no matter

342

how strong and healthy she appears to be. The wisdom of this is obvious from a comparison of the curability of cancer of the uterus in very early, moderately advanced, and late stages of disease. Treatment of very early cancer of the uterus will cure 75 per cent or more. About 40 per cent of the moderately advanced cases, which is the condition in which most women with the disease are first seen by the doctor, can be cured. And of the late and extensive cases, fewer than 10 per cent can be saved. If you have to have cancer of the cervix (and don't say it can't happen to you), which group do you chose to be in? The choice is yours—and wholly yours.

Cancer of the cervix seems to be more frequent among women who have borne children than among those who have not, and one explanation for this is that childbearing often causes tears or lacerations which if unrepaired result in chronic inflammatory conditions which the doctors call cervicitis. Inflammation and chronic infections of this organ can and often do have other causes, but the cause is beside the point, which is that all such abnormal conditions can be eliminated; and since they appear to favor the development of cancer, they should be.

LUNG

Cancer of the lung is rapidly becoming one of the commonest types of malignant tumor. Fifty years ago it was almost unheard of; twenty years ago it was rare; but today it is second only to the stomach as a cause of death from cancer, and a few observers believe that it may now be the most frequent of all the major forms of cancer. No other kind of cancer has shown so striking an increase.

Lung cancer is chiefly a disease of the male sex, twenty men being affected for every woman. The most constant first symptom is cough. As is the case of other signs and symptoms which have been noted, correct interpretation of cough is made difficult by the fact that so many people have coughs more or less continuously. Chronic bronchitis, sinus trouble, the widespread "cold" with a cough that hangs on for weeks or months, and the "cigarette cough" are so familiar in most temperate climates that the cough, like the cry of "wolf" sounded too often, excites nobody. The fact remains that cough is one of the first expressions of lung cancer, and so it deserves more respect than it gets. A cough of long standing, even if it can be proved to be due to causes other than cancer or tuberculosis, deserves respect for another reason. The usual chronic cough which is not caused by a tumor is usually the result of inflamed, irritated, perhaps infected membranes of the bronchial tubes. Possibly this state of irritation is a predisposing factor in the origin of cancer, and therefore should be eliminated always. Besides, a cough is a personal inconvenience and a social nuisance. But since coughs are such frequent aftermaths of the simple cold, when does one make the decision that the time has come to make certain that it is not due to a more serious condition? The safest rule is to investigate the source of any cough—no matter how logically it can be explained on a trivial basis—which persists undiminished for *three* weeks. This rule holds for the cough that hangs on following a chest cold, and for the cough of chronic bronchitis which has been present for years (because a diagnosis of chronic bronchitis or anything else does not confer immunity from cancer).

The cough of lung cancer sooner or later becomes productive of phlegm or sputum, the character of which is extremely varied. It may be frothy and colorless or thick and containing pus, and so there are no features of the expectoration which can be said to be typical of cancer, with the single exception of blood. Blood in the sputum, even in very small amounts—as fine streaks, for instance—can never be regarded lightly, and its appearance, even once, should always be reported to a physician. Another sign which presents fairly often in lung cancer and at a relatively early stage is a faint wheezing sound which accompanies breathing. It is not necessarily constant. The patient himself is usually the first to notice this faint sound and he may do so only when he is quiet and undistracted by other sounds. Somewhat later in the course of the disease chest pain appears. If infection develops in the tumor or in the portion of the lung being interfered with by the tumor, fever and night sweats occur. Loss of weight and weakness are present eventually.

But as has proved true for some other forms of cancer previously discussed, the "early" signs or symptoms of lung cancer are not necessarily early in the tumor's growth and course. This explains in part why the curative operation of pneumonectomy, surgical removal of the infected lung, can be undertaken in less than a fourth of the entire lung cancer group; the disease is too far advanced in the rest. But there is a simple, inexpensive, painless, and reliable "test" which will reveal the presence of tumors of the lung *before* they are large enough to produce cough or other symptoms. This test consists of an X-ray picture of the chest. Such films can disclose small and unsuspected tumors both benign and cancerous in the lungs of presumably perfectly healthy persons, as the recent experiences with large-scale chest X-ray surveys have shown. And the early returns on patients whose lung cancers have been found through routine chest X-rays—persons, remember, who seem to be in good health and without any complaints—suggest that the treatment at such a stage of disease will cure as high as 75 per cent—or more than three times as many as can be cured once the symptoms have developed. This immensely important fact is all the proof that any sane man or woman should need as to the value of the routine chest X-ray twice a year beyond the age of fifty. (Lung cancer is extremely rare before then.) The first human being ever operated on successfully for cancer of the lung is living and carrying on an active medical practice nineteen years later, and since that historic operation was performed this has been a potentially curable disease. But only a fraction of this potential has been achieved up to now—and the reason is again—too late. The little time and cost of a chest film is a small premium indeed to pay for so large a measure of protection against needless, avoidable death.

Much has been heard in late years of virus pneumonia. It so happens that it seems to occur with surprising frequency in patients with cancer of the lung—and early in the course of the cancer at that. It is not uncommon for X-rays, taken in order to diagnose an acute infection of the lung—virus pneumonia, for example—to disclose an unsuspected lung cancer. But sometimes the area of pneumonia overlies or surrounds the cancer so as to hide it in the X-ray picture; therefore, it is highly important that X-rays of the chest be taken several weeks after recovery from virus pneumonia in order to be perfectly sure that evidence of infection as disclosed in the X-ray has disappeared as it should, and that no lurking cancer continues to cast its shadow.

Until very recently many theories had been advanced to explain the appalling increase in lung cancer over the last thirty years. One theory which received wide medical attention was that the rise in cigarette consumption was related to the increase in lung cancer. In 1964 this theory became a proven fact when the United States Government officially announced that a definite causative link exists between lung cancer and other major diseases and heavy cigarette smoking. After fourteen months of studying all available medical evidence the U.S. Surgeon General's Office warned that continued use of tobacco was harmful to health. Smoking was linked with pulmonary, heart and circulatory ailments as well as with lung cancer.

Inhalation of certain dusts or fumes generated in particular industrial operations is a proven hazard in respect of lung cancer causation, and other dusts and fumes are suspected. The fumes from anthracene oil, chromates, and nickel carbonyl are factors in cancer of the lung. However, most occupational dangers are recognized, and workers are protected by proper hygienic regulations.

BLADDER

Cancer of the bladder is given special mention here, not because it is especially frequent but because of the universal neglect of its early warning signs, which is largely responsible for the present poor results of treatment. Blood in the urine is the most important—in fact, the only—early signal of bladder cancer. It may first appear in several successive urinations, or it may appear but once. Usually there is a somewhat extended interval, amounting to weeks or months before it is seen again. During this period of freedom from bleeding, the alarm with which the patient reacted to the first shocking appearance of blood in his urine gives way to hopefulness that it won't happen again and, as time goes on, to varying degrees of assurance that it will not, but, soon or late —there it is again! The average patient—it is more often a man—delays six and one half months after he first passes bloody urine before telling his doctor about it. Blood in the urine does not always mean cancer, but cancer is the most important thing it can mean, and immediate investigation of the genital and urinary organs is called for. A single episode of bloody urine is enough to not wait for a second.

TESTICLE

Tumors of the testicle are rather rare—yet because they occur almost exclusively in young men in their twenties, with life before them, they are especially important to recognize. A life saved at this age means many more years of living than a life saved at fifty or sixty. There are but two signs calling attention to growths in the testicle: one is enlargement, so that one testis looks and feels bigger than its mate; the second is increase in density, so that the testicle in which the tumor is present feels heavier than its mate and this heaviness may be noted by the patient as a "dragging sensation." Most varieties of testicular tumors spread quickly, making the earliest possible treatment essential.

PROSTATE

Cancer of the prostate is probably the commonest cancer affecting men. It does not appear as the first cause of male cancer deaths simply because in many cases it is not diagnosed. This is understandable when it is realized that quite often the disease runs a slow, chronic course, and even when present may not be the primary cause of death and may not even give rise to symptoms. Yet prostatic cancer is responsible for some 10 per cent of cancer deaths in men, being third among the causes of such deaths. Cancer of the prostate may produce two quite different kinds of first symptoms. One kind, due to the enlargement of the prostate itself, consists of urinary difficulty of one sort or another. The other is pain in other parts of the body, for instance in the lower spine, resulting from spread of the disease to the bones of the skeleton. Thus symptoms may be local or general and, of course, both may be present together. The local symptoms—difficulty in urinating—often begin as a narrowing of the stream and a lessening of its force. Dribbling after urination becomes annoying. Later, as the prostate grows larger, it is necessary to force the urine out by contracting the abdominal muscles. Eventually complete obstruction may occur. If the tumor grows into the urinary passage or the base of the bladder, blood may appear in the urine. These signs are not necessarily proof of prostatic cancer, for they can also be caused by benign enlargement of that organ, termed hypertrophy, which is so common in elderly males. However, the possibility of cancer is so strong that immediate medical consultation should be sought at the first evidence of urinary irregularity. Certain cancers of the prostate remain relatively small within the prostate itself even while spreading by metastasis to other parts of the body—the bones usually. This explains why a man with no significant urinary symptoms may develop pains in the back or hip or neck and be found to have deposits of tumors scattered through the bones, as shown in X-ray pictures. As with all other kinds of cancer, cure is possible only when the disease is found to be localized, although, as will be seen, remarkable restraint of the growth, amounting sometimes to control, can often be achieved.

There is one way to discover cancer of the prostate at a time when it is localized and can be entirely removed; it is the periodic, twice yearly examination of the prostate of every man over fifty. This is a simple doctor's office procedure consisting of carefully feeling the prostate through the rectum. Actually examination of the rectum and prostate is performed at one and the same time. Even very small prostatic tumors can be felt in this way—still too small to cause any symptoms. The discovery of prostate cancer before it produces symptoms gives the patient an excellent chance of cure, and in view of the prevalence of this disease, no intelligent man can fail to concede the value of this form of life assurance—the regular examination of his supposedly normal prostate. Although surgical removal of the prostate while the disease is contained in that structure is the only means of effecting a cure, within the past few years it has become possible to greatly prolong the lives and relieve the discomfort of patients with widespread metastatic prostate cancer, and in some cases this growth restraint has amounted to a long-lasting arrest of the disease. This effect is achieved by castration or by the administration of female sex hormones or by both. Treated in this fashion, men with cancer of the prostate who a few years ago could expect to live no more than a year or a year and a half can now look forward to living twice that long, and, most important of all, in comparative comfort.

BONE

Malignant tumors of bone (bone sarcoma) are rather rare, but like tumors of the testicle their tendency to occur in young people from five to twenty years old makes them important. When the tumor arising in a bone grows large enough, it will appear as a swelling. Many bone tumors, especially malignant ones, are apt to develop at the ends of bones, near joints, and because of this motion of the joint may be interfered with fairly early—to a degree which causes slight disability or discomfort. Thus a tumor growing near the knee or hip may have the effect of limiting the normal movement of the adjacent joints so that a slight limp may be produced. Malignant tumors of bone constitute a notable exception to the generality that pain is not an early symptom of cancer. Pain is apt to occur early in bone sarcoma, and it tends to occur at night or to be worse at night. Swelling, mild dysfunction, and pain, then, are the signs of importance in bone tumors.

LYMPHOMAS

A large class of malignant tumorlike diseases differs from those which have been presented thus far in that they do not usually arise in one organ or site, but rather in entire systems or widely scattered parts of systems. Leukemia is a good example of diseases of this type, arising as it does in the blood-forming tissues of the body, notably the bone marrow, the spleen, and the lymph glands. Hodgkin's disease is another, originating in deposits of lymphoid tissue —the lymph glands. The lymphatic apparatus is also involved in lymphosarcoma, another of the generalized malignant tumors. The unique feature of diseases of this class is that they tend to be systematized or generalized from the beginning. There are exceptions to this, for occasionally lymphosarcoma appears as a localized lesion and has been treated successfully under such circumstances. However, Hodgkin's disease and usually lymphosarcoma are prone to involve multiple areas, with the lymph glands of the neck, armpit, groin, abdomen, and mid-chest (mediastinum) as the usual sites. At first the disease may seem to be restricted to the nodes of a single area, and thus be localized to some extent. The first evidence of either of these disorders is an enlarged or swollen lymph gland or several such. These initially large nodes are seen more often in the neck than anywhere else. Lymph node enlargement without obvious infection to account for it should be laid before the doctor, who may decide after reviewing all the evidence to remove the node in question in order to be certain of its nature.

Doctors of a few generations ago had a striking term for leukemia—"flowing cancer." It is thought of as a kind of cancer of the blood, and is fully discussed with blood diseases. While a tumor in the usual sense is not present, still the overproduction of white blood cells is a growth irregularity which is fundamentally similar to the cellular processes of cancer. In the case of leukemia the white cells are released into the volume of circulating blood. The number of white cells is sometimes very high (300,000 per cubic millimeter as compared with the normal 8,000), but sometimes the number is only moderately increased and occasionally it may be below normal. The age of the white blood cells, that is, their degree of maturity, is a more reliable basis for diagnosing and following the progress of leukemia than the actual number of blood cells. Leukemia may make itself known in a number of ways. The spleen or lymph nodes may enlarge and first call attention to illness. There may be an increased tendency to bleed, with troublesome oozing from gums or spontaneous small hemorrhages into the skin showing as small, perfectly flat, circular, rose-purple areas. A number of cases are diagnosed in consequence of persistent bleeding following the extraction of a tooth. Leukemia is usually associated with some degree of anemia; hence there may be pallor, fatigue, and shortness of breath. Most often the earliest symptoms are extremely vague, and patients will complain of little except not feeling up to par. Leukemia may be acute—running through its natural untreated course in a matter of weeks—or chronic, lasting for several years and showing alternating periods of activity and remission, the latter induced by treatment, or now and then occurring spontaneously. Patients with chronic leukemia can be kept quite comfortable and active, their lives perhaps prolonged, through judicious use of X-ray treatment and more recently, in selected cases, radioactive isotopes and a few chemical agents such as the nitrogen mustard compounds. Until three years ago there was no treatment which had any effect on acute leukemia, but through the administration of ACTH or cortisone and certain newly discovered chemical compounds called folic acid antagonists, it is now possible to induce significant regression of disease in up to two thirds of the young patients. (Acute leukemia is almost wholly a disease of children.) Hodgkin's disease and lymphosarcoma are usually managed for several years by carefully applied X-rays—and in later stages certain new drugs (nitrogen mustard compounds, triethylenemelamine, and others) prove useful in maintaining the patient in comfort.

CHILDHOOD

Cancer in children is rare, and yet it is an important cause of death in childhood, certainly more important than many of the usual childhood diseases. In fact, cancer causes more deaths between the ages of five and fourteen than any other disease. (Accidents lead the mortality table in this age group—accounting for one third of all deaths at this period of life.)

Cancers of all types occur in children, but sarcomas far outnumber carcinomas. Certain malignant tumors appear almost exclusively before the age of ten. In rare instances babies have been born with cancer. The organs and systems which are the usual sites of malignant tumors appearing in children are the eye; kidney; bones; lymph nodes; throat; nerve structures, including the brain, and soft peripheral parts such as muscle. All that has been said about the tendency of early cancer to imitate or resemble many benign and trivial conditions applies even more to young children, because the confusion is confounded by their inability to express themselves fully.

The commoner signs of the commoner malignant tumors of childhood are (1) a gray, greenish, or milky-white glint seen in the eye—in the presence of a tumor arising in the nerves of the posterior portion of the eye, (2) swelling seen or felt in the abdomen caused by tumor of the kidney or of the nerve tissues in the region of the kidney, (3) pain in an extremity worse at night, with or without associated swelling—suggesting bone tumor, (4) enlargement of the glands or bleeding tendencies, with or without small rose or violet discolorations in the skin, indicating the possibility of Hodgkin's disease, lymphosarcoma, or leukemia, (5) difficulty in swallowing or in breathing (causing audible breath sounds), pointing to tumors of the throat or chest, (6) persistent cough which steadily gets worse, caused by tumors within the chest, (7) stomach and intestinal symptoms not accounted for by infection or by inflammation within the alimentary tract, due to tumors of the nervous system (brain and sympathetic nerve structures), (8) continuing unexplained fever, (9) tiredness, lack of interest, decrease of appetite and loss of weight which persist beyond a reasonable period, say a week or ten days. The kinds of cancer which typically affect children seem to show unusually rapid growth. In general, treatment of them is not nearly so successful as the treatment of cancer in adults. Early recognition of the real causes of the complaints and abnormal signs in young patients offers the only hope of improving the results. It should be observed once more that cancer is rare in children, and no parent is justified in worrying about it nor in being oversolicitous in trying to interpret the early evidences of the usual childhood ills which can be quite perplexing. A reasonable rule would be to rely on the *duration* of any departure from normal. Because the great majority of children's affections are acute, developing quickly, running a relatively rapid course, and subsiding quickly, any mild evidence of illness or abnormality which lasts beyond ten days—even though it does not appear serious—should be presented to the doctor.

Many kinds of cancer have been omitted from this discussion. Most of the growths which have not been described are rare. Finally, for most of the tumors omitted, the factor of early diagnosis appears to be of less critical importance in determining the outcome than is the case for most of those which have been described. As examples of the tumors in this category, the following may be cited: (1) Tumors of the brain and spinal cord, whose signs—extremely diverse, depending upon the location of the lesion—include disturbances of sight (such as double vision), loss of balance, weakness, and paralysis of certain muscle groups and tremors. (2) Malignant tumors of muscles, tendons and the like, called soft part sarcomas. Here the sole sign which could possibly be of assistance in speeding the patient toward diagnosis is a swelling—that is the presence of a tumor mass. (3) Cancers arising in organs which are not removable or removable with great risk, such as the liver and pancreas. (4) Miscellaneous cancers such as those of the thyroid gland (a solitary lump in the neck or a goiter-like swelling), kidney, ovary, and so on.

RESEARCH

Many people believe that not very much is known about cancer and that not much progress is being made toward discovering its causes. On the contrary, probably more facts are known about cancer than about any other disease, although still not enough to provide effective means of control. Almost all that is known has come in the past fifty years, and still more encouraging is the fact that cancer research is now expanding rapidly—indeed, on the basis of cost, it

Cancer — One of the great hopes in cancer research is chemotherapy, a chemical means of destroying cancer cells without injuring the patient. This scientist is checking up on a laboratory experiment that may provide clues in the unending search for cures for cancer.

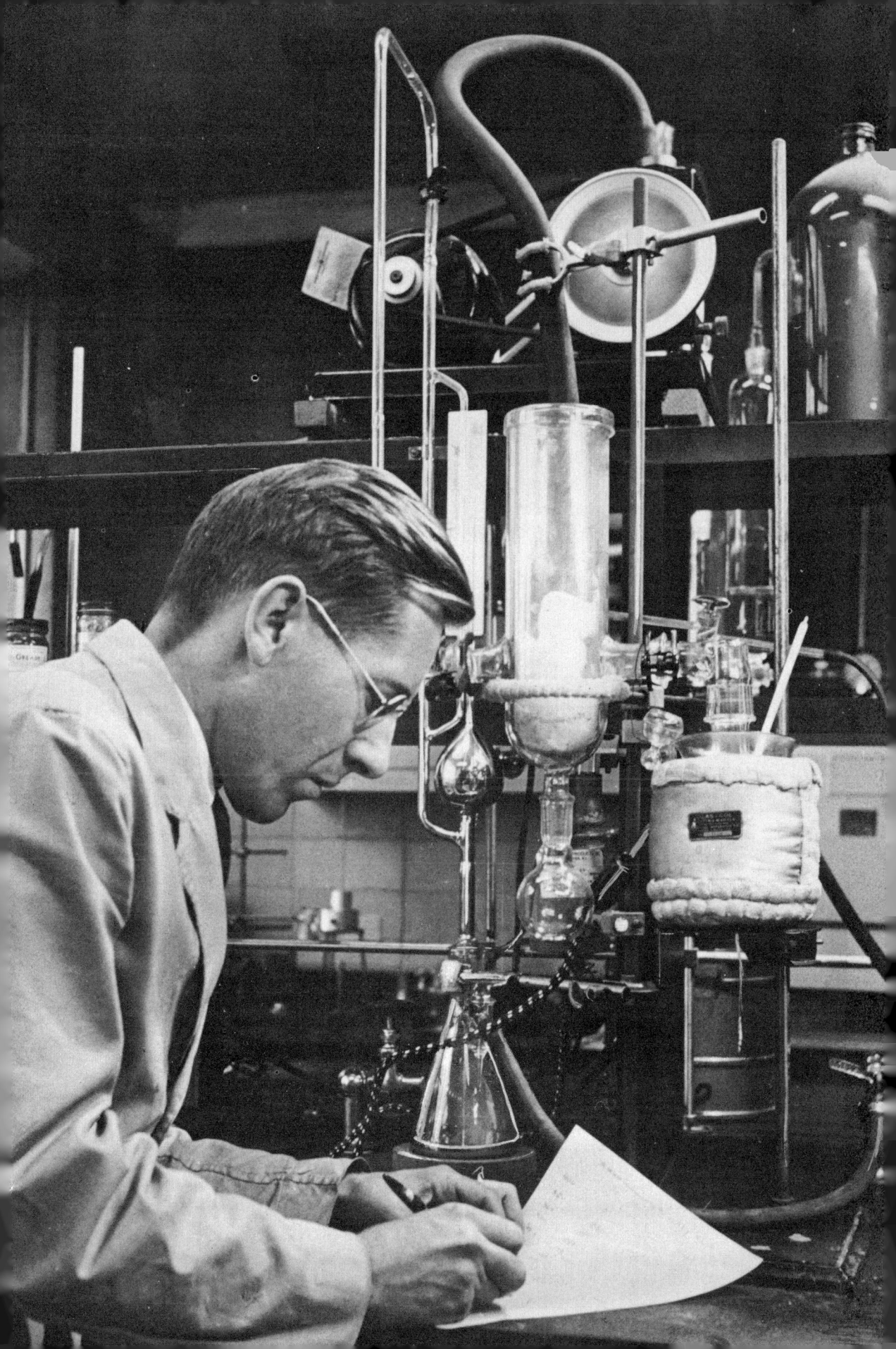

has increased twelvefold in the past ten years and now amounts to about fifteen million dollars annually in the United States alone.

Research has disclosed evidence that for certain cancer in animals heredity is a factor. It has been possible by selective breeding to "bring out" cancer susceptibility in mice, for instance, so that almost every female will develop it, and conversely, the cancer tendency can be overcome by breeding so that resistant strains are established in which it never appears. Since heredity appears to be governed by the structure called genes, found in the nucleus of cells, much research attention is now directed at the gene and how it works. But the tendency to cancer in mice is evidently not wholly dependent on genes, because it has recently been shown that if the newborn offspring of cancer-susceptible parents are prevented from nursing at their own mother's breast and placed instead with foster nurses of a cancer-resistant breed, they will not get breast cancer as expected. Evidently breast milk is also a factor, and later studies suggest that it contains a virus which may be the cancer inciter. There is no clear evidence that such a factor influences human breast cancer, nor for any other kind of human cancer, although viruses are responsible for four kinds of cancer occurring in the rabbit, frog, and mouse. Genetic influences may also be modified by removing the ovaries of infant females of cancer-susceptible breeds; and cancer can be made to develop in the offspring of resistant strains by giving them large doses of female sex hormones. As noted previously, the course of cancer originating in certain organs controlled by sex hormones, as the prostate and breast, can usually be modified by altering the hormone pattern. This is done by castration and administering the proper hormone. The importance of hormones in cancer is also shown in the recent discovery that the make-up of hormones (as revealed in the way they are excreted in the urine) is different in cancer patients as compared to healthy persons. About 350 chemical compounds are known which will cause cancer under controlled conditions of the research laboratory, and efforts are under way to find out just how they convert the normal cell to a cancerous one, and whether any such chemicals can be "accidentally" formed by the body itself.

If, as has been said, life is a continuous series of chemical reactions, then so must cancer be. Up to now it has not been possible to analyze the chemistry of the body in minute detail, but recently developed machines and methods now are doing it. Radioactive isotopes enable the scientist to trace the fate of many substances within the body; microscopes of greater power than any used before and other physical equipment now permit determination of the chemical structure of the smallest parts of cells, and exploration of the complex changes which are the basis of life and growth and, very likely, cancer. Once these are understood, it is reasonable to expect that ways can be found to alter the chemistry of cancer, interrupting the chain of reactions leading to abnormal cell growth and setting the chemical balance to rights. Already under way is an intensive search for chemical compounds which will seek out cancer cells and destroy them, without harming normal tissues. Several such chemotherapy agents have been found which partially fulfil these requirements, not sufficiently, however, to destroy all the cancer cells in a given tumor. The most useful are derivatives of nitrogen mustard gas of wartime development, and the anti-folic compounds, which prevent the cells' use of folic acid, a vitamin which rapidly dividing cells need in large quantity.

Thus the general objectives of cancer research are to learn more about the causes of abnormal growth so that cancer may ultimately be prevented, and to find more effective methods of treating it, once it has occurred. From these brief references to research, it will be seen that cancer appears to be due to not just one cause, and it is quite possible that no one preventive or treatment method will prove effective for all tumors. As is always the way of science, each experiment undertaken opens up new paths to be explored, so that the opportunities for further research are increasing year by year. Sooner or later the great mass of information now being assembled will begin to assume meaning, and the outline of the picture we are seeking will gradually appear—not all of a sudden, but as the pieces of a jigsaw puzzle fall into place—bit by bit.

GOAL

Fortunately, it is not necessary to wait for research to forge the final answers to cancer in order to achieve a significantly larger measure of control over this disease than we now have. If present knowledge were to be fully put to use, if all cancer were to be treated within weeks instead of within months, as is the case generally, twice as many lives could be saved as are now being saved. The core of the problem of present-day cancer control is early treatment, and if it is to be achieved on a wide scale, the public must recognize that its responsibility is hardly less than that of the doctors. Your responsibility is twofold. First you must learn that you will be the first to receive the initial expressions of cancer and you must therefore prepare yourself for this possibility (a good possibility since cancer will affect one in every five now living) by learning its Seven Danger Signals. But it is now possible to forestall the appearance of certain of these danger signals and by the many months saved to increase greatly the chances of successful treatment. Methods are at hand for finding cancer in certain organs long before it would normally cause signs or symptoms, and these methods are simple, inexpensive, and applicable on a broad scale. Your second responsibility, then, is to take advantage of these cancer-detecting procedures by having a careful physical examination at regular intervals—no matter how fit you feel. Experience has proven that cancer may and does exist long before it calls attention to its presence—yet it can be found IF it is looked for. This is particularly true of cancer of the lung, womb, breast, and rectum, because of the ease with which these sites can be examined at proper intervals. The general physical examination including these organs and also an X-ray picture of the chest should be as routine for women over thirty-five and men over forty-five as the periodic visit to the dentist has become. It is likely to be a lot less painful, too.

The periodic health checkup has been advocated by doctors for years, but relatively few people have taken advantage of it. Its importance is increasing, however, because it offers the only means of coping with diseases which have now become our leading health problems owing to longer life. It is not possible to deal with cancer and high blood pressure and hardening of the arteries as the previous major health menaces have been dealt with. They are not controllable by vaccination or quarantine, by regulation of sewage disposal or water purification. There are no wonder drugs to combat them, no vitamins to build resistance against them. Instead, the responsibility for their control is squarely up to every man and woman, and it cannot be transferred to anyone else nor to any agency. Acceptance or rejection of this responsibility will largely determine how much farther the span of life can be lengthened—our life as a people and our lives as individuals.

CANCER, TREATMENT OF. The treatment of cancer differs in one fundamental respect from that of most other diseases. The cure for most other diseases is accomplished by the body itself; the treatment consists of creating favorable conditions for this self-help. In cancer, however, the body defenses are helpless. Not only is the body unable to destroy the growth but actually it may nourish the cancer at the expense of the healthy organs and tissues. The successful treatment of cancer is one which eliminates or destroys all the cancer cells with as little harm as possible to the healthy cells and tissues of the body.

The only means now available for curing cancer are surgery and radiation. If a cancer is detected early enough—that is, when it is still localized and has not spread—such treatment has proved extremely valuable. However, the more advanced the cancer when treatment is started, the less likely is cure. Developments in surgical and radiation therapy combined with early diagnosis have, without doubt, increased the cure rate. Unfortunately treatment of widespread cancer has not been successful. This has led to much research and an intensive search for chemicals, including hormones, which can seek out and destroy cancer cells anywhere in the body in a manner similar to the way in which antibiotics destroy bacteria.

Surgery has been and still remains the most widely used treatment for cancer and has resulted in the highest percentage of cures. The chance for cure is highest when the cancer is removed while still localized or confined to the tissue or organ where it developed. Cancers which have spread to the surrounding area may be removed by more extensive (called radical) surgery, such as that of the breast in which the lymph nodes in the armpit are also removed. Better pre- and postoperative management of the patient as well as improved surgical techniques and antibiotics have improved the value and effectiveness of surgical treatment.

Radiation therapy is not of equal value in the treatment of all cancers. Cancers vary greatly in their response to such treatment. For some cancers, such as those of the skin, lip, and cervix, irradiation may be the treatment of choice, giving better results than surgery. In others, both methods are equally suitable. Still others should be treated only by surgery. In still other cases, radiation therapy is used in conjunction with surgery as a pre- and postoperative treatment.

With the recent development of new multimillion-volt x-ray generators and radioactive Cobalt-60, many cancers deep within the body which were not previously within the range of radiation therapy may be treated. Better techniques have made possible the more effective treatment of the cancer with less damage to the surrounding tissue.

The injection into the body of radioactive isotopes has made possible the treatment of certain widespread cancers. For example, radioactive iodine not only destroys some thyroid cancers but can also seek out metastatic spread of these cancers throughout the body and eliminate them. Radioactive phosphorus has been used to treat cancer of the lymphatic system. Radioactive gold has been used in the treatment of prostate cancer.

Hormonal therapy is used in the treatment of widespread cancers of the breast and prostate because these organs are influenced by hormones, which are internal secretions of the ductless glands. Treatment consists of removal of the sex and occasionally adrenal glands in order to remove the source of the hormones which stimulate the growth of these cancers. Such treatment also makes use of female sex hormones to neutralize the male sex hormones in the case of prostate cancer, and the use of male sex hormones in the treatment of premenopausal women with breast cancer, and female sex hormones in the treatment of postmenopausal women. In some cases, like expectancy has been increased as much as a year.

By *chemotherapy* is meant the treatment of cancer with chemicals which can identify, seek out, and destroy malignant cells and tissues but which will not harm surrounding normal healthy tissues. Because cancer cells differ from normal cells— as demonstrated by their relatively uncontrollable wild growth—they probably differ in their food requirements. This observation led to the possibility of discovering chemicals or drugs which can selectively starve or poison cancer cells. This idea is similar to that involved in the control of bacterial infection by antibiotics. Although cancers have not been generally cured by drugs alone, some chemotherapeutic substances have been useful in easing or eliminating pain and prolonging life. They have been particularly useful in treatment of leukemia and Hodgkin's disease. Among these drugs being used are nitrogen mustard, 6-Mercaptopurine, methotrexate, and two long-named chemicals abbreviated as TEM and TEPA. *See also* CANCER.

CANKER SORE, usually a small ulceration on the inside of the mouth, lips, and cheeks, which may appear from a variety of causes. Sometimes the cause stems from the nervous system; often the sore is a manifestation of a sensitivity to certain substances taken into the body; and frequently it is due to a virus infection such as a cold. Whenever canker sores appear persistently, a medical study should be made for some functional disturbance, including an examination of the blood to determine the status of the clotting elements in the blood stream. Tests should also be made for sensitivity to various foods, and the fillings in the patient's teeth examined, since it has been shown that dissimilar metals used as fillings in the same mouth may create electrical currents sometimes associated with the appearance of cankers in the mouth.

CANTHARIDES, popularly called

Spanish fly, a bitter-tasting powder made from an insect known scientifically as Cantharis vasicatoria. The active principle in the drug is cantharidin, which is marketed in many forms, such as cantharidin plaster, blistering fluid, cantharidin ointment, and tincture of cantharidin.

The drug should be used only when prescribed by a doctor, and the utmost precaution should be taken to prevent it from entering the mouth, the eyes, or other sensitive areas.

Cantharidin is never used before the condition of the patient's kidneys has been checked, since the drug is easily absorbed through the skin. It must not be applied to any part of the body on which the patient is likely to lie, since the heat and perspiration result in blistering. Furthermore, it is dangerous when applied to paralyzed arms or legs. Such reputation as it has as a stimulant to sexual desire is without any good evidence.

Cantharides is intensely irritating to the kidneys and should never be taken internally. In the treatment of children, the aged, or the weak it should never be used, even externally, for any purpose.

Symptoms of cantharidin poisoning may be intense pain in the alimentary canal, in the stomach and kidneys, or in the urinary organs. Vomiting and diarrhea ordinarily occur, and a persistent desire to urinate is noticeable. The pulse is usually weak and slow and collapse is not unlikely. *See also* BLISTERS.

CANTHARIDES—poisoning: See article FIRST AID, page 830.

CAPILLARIES, the smallest branches of the arterial tree; fine, filament-like vessels through which blood pumped by the heart through increasingly smaller branches of the arterial tree finally passes by osmosis, an exchange of substances, to the cells of body organs and tissues. They are the minute structural elements which connect arterial circulation with venous circulation and which carry deoxygenated blood back to the heart. *See also* BLOOD; CIRCULATORY SYSTEM.

CAPILLARIES – See articles BLOOD PRESSURE, page 244; THE SKIN, page 1723.

CAPILLARIES – lung: See article DISEASES OF THE HEART AND CIRCULATION, page 983-84.

CARBOHYDRATES, organic substances which contain carbon, hydrogen, and oxygen and are stable, easily digestible sources of calories or nutritional energy. They belong to the class of nutriments represented by sugars, starches, celluloses, and gums. Foods with large carbohydrate content are sugars, jams, jellies, preserves, syrups, molasses, honey, cocoa, chocolate, candy, grains, grain products, and farinaceous substances. Nuts, although they contain a larger proportion per weight of protein, and an even greater proportion of fats, are also substantial in carbohydrate content. All dairy products, fruits and vegetables have carbohydrates in varying amounts. Dates and figs are especially rich in this nutriment, and potatoes, parsnips, and most lentils are also plentifully supplied with carbohydrates. *See also* NUTRITION.

CARBOHYDRATES – amount in common foods: See article DIABETES, page 546.

CARBON DIOXIDE, a colorless odorless gas, a molecule of which consists of one atom of carbon in combination with two atoms of oxygen. It is one of the end products of the cellular metabolism of proteins, carbohydrates, and fats, all of which are carbon-containing compounds. It is given off by the body during that phase of respiration known as exhalation. The oxygen taken in during inhalation passes through the walls of capillaries lining the lungs, combines with the iron in the red blood corpuscles, is carried to the heart and from there distributed by the arterial system to all the cells of the body. In these cells, together with other substances, it enters into the chemical reactions essential to life. The carbon dioxide,

among other waste products which result, passes through the cell walls into the venous blood supply, back to the heart, and from there to the lungs where it is exhaled. Although residual amounts in the blood stream are essential for normal body function, carbon dioxide in sufficient concentration can cause death. Generally the amount of this gas contained in the atmosphere is less than .03 per cent. In an unventilated room crowded with people, the concentration might rise dangerously. An atmospheric concentration of about 25 per cent is said to be lethal, but symptoms of a rising carbon dioxide concentration, such as headaches and drowsiness, would set in much earlier. In cities, carbon dioxide concentration is increased by the combustion of carbon-containing compounds in transportation, heating, and industrial processes. Fortunately urban atmospheres are continuously refreshed by winds which carry oxygen-laden air to the city and dust and carbon dioxide-laden air from it. The presence of green plants also helps decrease the carbon dioxide content of atmosphere, since plants predominantly inhale carbon dioxide and exhale oxygen during the process of photosynthesis. This takes place during sunlight; and at night, like the human being, the plant takes in small quantities of oxygen for its cellular metabolism and gives off some carbon dioxide as waste. Throughout a twenty-four-hour period, however, the plant removes much more carbon dioxide than oxygen, and gives off much more oxygen than carbon dioxide.

CARBON MONOXIDE, a colorless odorless gas, a product of the incomplete combustion of carbon. It is extremely poisonous. It burns with a pale blue flame to form carbon dioxide. Carbon monoxide may develop when coal oil, charcoal, gas, or kerosene are burned in a poorly ventilated room. A frequent source of carbon monoxide is from the exhausts of automobiles. In the open air, the gas quickly becomes carbon dioxide, but in a closed garage a running motor may produce enough carbon monoxide to kill in a matter of minutes.

Carbon monoxide invades the blood stream through the lungs, unites with the hemoglobin in the red blood corpuscles so that they cannot carry oxygen to the cells of the body, and asphyxiation ensues. The blood of victims of carbon-monoxide poisoning is a bright cherry red.

Early symptoms of carbon-monoxide poisoning include yawning, headache, nausea, dizziness, ringing in the ears, and abdominal pains. Gaspy breathing and unconsciousness quickly follow. The victim should get fresh air immediately, and he should be kept lying down and warm. A physician should be called promptly, and inhalations of oxygen or of oxygen-carbon dioxide mixture administered. Pure oxygen accelerates the release of carbon monoxide and frees it from the blood about four times faster than simple inhalation of air. If the breathing of the victim is gasping or has stopped, artificial respiration should be given at once.

If the carbon-monoxide poisoning is serious, the victim should be taken to the hospital as soon as possible for treatment which may include blood transfusions. Since the nerve cells are involved in the poisoning, temporary or permanent damage can be done to the brain, with serious disturbances of vision, hearing, speech, and memory.

Because carbon monoxide cannot be seen or smelled, danger of poisoning is especially insidious. Care should be taken that rooms in which fuels capable of producing carbon monoxide are being burned are properly ventilated, and that a car motor is not kept running in a closed garage.

CARBON MONOXIDE — sewer gas: See article OCCUPATION AND HEALTH, page 1383.

CARBUNCLES, painful infections of the skin layer below the surface, accompanied by the production and discharge of pus and dead tissue, and tending to affect the general health. A carbuncle may be distinguished from a boil by its greater severity and depth and especially by its having several openings instead of one.

The first symptom of a carbuncle is a painful hard lump which develops under a tight and reddening skin. Several pus-discharging openings later appear in this surface. Eventually the entire mass will tend to separate itself, leaving an open sore.

Carbuncles appear most frequently on the face, neck, and shoulders. They particularly afflict persons who suffer from diabetes or Bright's disease. In such people resistance to invasive microorganisms which set up infection is lowered.

The severity of the infection can often be diminished at the outset by means of x-ray treatment, sulfa drugs, or penicillin. The immediate pain may be relieved by the application of hot compresses. These increase the flow of blood, thus strengthening the defensive forces in the infected area.

When the accumulation of pus becomes considerable, the carbuncle should be opened and drained by a physician. Unless special precautions are taken during this operation the protective wall, which the tissues have built to seal the infection from the rest of the body, may be broken down, thus permitting the infection to spread.

To avoid a repetition of this painful and exhausting experience, the person should have himself tested for diabetes and Bright's disease which predispose the body to this type of infection. The person should pay increased attention to the state of his general health; the body must develop resistance against such invasion. *See also* FURUNCLES.

CARBUNCLES — See article THE SKIN, page 1761-62.
CARBUNCLES — occupational incidence: See article OCCUPATION AND HEALTH, page 1359.
CARBUNCLES — scalp: See article THE HAIR, page 959.
CARBUNCLES — wet dressings: See article THE SKIN, page 1742.

CARCINOGENS, substances or agents that cause the development of cancer of any type—for example, certain tar or coal products.

CARDIAC AND CORONARY. The word "cardiac" is frequently used as an adjective to replace the word "heart"; for example, cardiac disease, cardiac pain, cardiac accidents. The word "coronary," which is used to describe the blood vessels that supply the heart with its blood and oxygen is associated also with other words to describe what may happen to the coronary artery. Thus, "coronary sclerosis" is a hardening of the coronary arteries; "coronary thrombosis" is a blocking of the coronary arteries, and anything abnormal about the coronary arteries or their function is

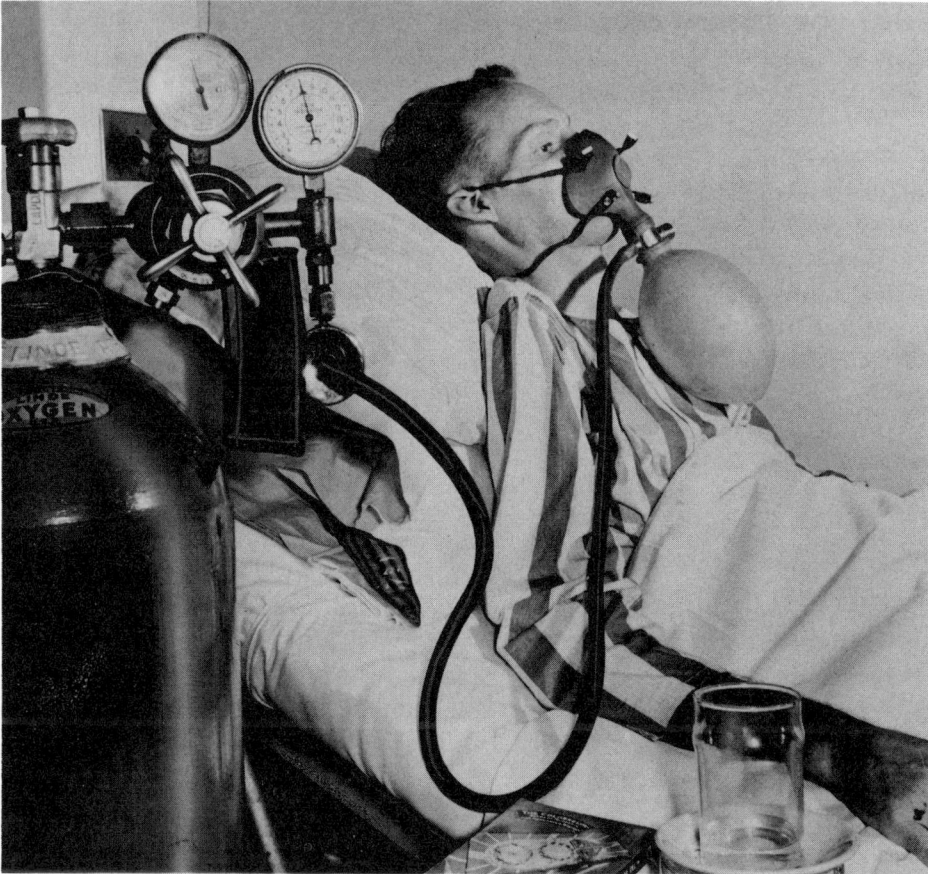

Cardiac and Coronary — One of the methods of treating the cardiac patient is the administration of oxygen. Oxygen helps the patient to breathe easier and relieves the heart of much of its burden.   *Three Lions, Inc.*

called "coronary disease." When a blood vessel is closed by the formation of a blood clot, as in coronary thrombosis, the muscles of the heart are suddenly deprived of their blood supply. The area that is thus deprived of blood will not be able to carry on its work and the tissues begin to break down and degenerate. This is called "coronary infarction." The area that does not have any blood is called an "infarct." Eventually healing occurs if

the person lives and a scar replaces the damaged tissue.

The various tissues of the heart are described according to their position as "endocardium" which is the lining of the heart; "pericardium" which is the sac which surrounds the heart; "myocardium" which is the muscle of the heart. *See also* CORONARY THROMBOSIS; HEART.

CARDITIS, an inflammation of the

heart, a manifestation and significant part of rheumatic fever. Internal carditis or endocarditis is the inflammation of the valves of the heart and membranes which line it. Pericarditis is the inflammation of the sac which encloses the heart. *See also* BACTERIAL ENDOCARDITIS; ENDOCARDITIS; PERICARDITIS.

CARDITIS – See article DISEASES OF THE HEART AND CIRCULATION, page 992-98.

CARDITIS – pericarditis: See articles DISEASES OF THE HEART AND CIRCULATION, page 994; THE KIDNEY: ITS DISEASES AND DISTURBANCES, page 1184-85.

CARMINATIVE, an agent which relieves flatulence and colic.

CAROTENE, a chemical precursor of vitamin A, is a yellow pigment found in green and yellow vegetables such as carrots, sweet potatoes, yellow corn, and string beans. It can be extracted in a chemical laboratory and is converted in the animal body into vitamin A. *See also* VITAMINS.

CAROTENE – See article DEFICIENCY DISEASES, page 500-01.

CAROTENE – in infant's diet: See article CARE AND FEEDING OF THE CHILD, page 1412.

CARPAL BONES, the eight bones of the wrist. On the back of the hand, five metacarpal bones connect the fingers with the wrist.

CARSICKNESS. *See* MOTION SICKNESS.

CARRIER OF DISEASE, the agent which transmits a communicable disease. It can be any of a vast number of things—air and dust, nose and throat secretions, sputum, clothing, insects. For example, certain mosquitoes carry malaria, dengue, and filariasis. Disease-producing bacteria cannot penetrate unbroken skin and must enter by means of wounds, scratches, abrasions, or a natural opening of the body. *See also* BACTERIA; INFECTIOUS DISEASES.

CARRIER OF DISEASE – See article THE PREVENTION AND TREATMENT OF INFECTIOUS DISEASE, page 1093-94.

CARRIER OF DISEASE – control: See article THE PREVENTION AND TREATMENT OF INFECTIOUS DISEASE, page 1096-97.

CARTILAGE, a white, semi-opaque connective tissue characterized by extreme smoothness, elasticity, and toughness. It covers the ends of the bones where they meet to become joints. Circular discs of cartilage lie, for example, between each layer of bone in the spine, acting as cushions or shock absorbers for these bones and for the strain to which the spinal column is subjected. Cartilage covers the movable joints of the legs, arms, and fingers, giving smoothness and resiliency to their movements. It is also found in other parts of the body, such as the tip of the nose, eyelids, ears, and the windpipe.

CARTILAGE – See article ENDOCRINOLOGY, page 708-09.

CARTILAGE – rickets: See article CARE AND FEEDING OF THE CHILD, page 1448.

CASCARA, a drug usually derived from the bark of a tree native to Mexico, and also from certain shrubs. Because of its effective action on the colon, cascara is widely used as a laxative. Usually cascara is prescribed in the form of an aromatic extract. Cascara sagrada, the bark of California buckthorn, is especially useful in cases of chronic constipation.

362

CASEIN, the principal protein in milk. In milk, a liquid precursor, caseinogen, is present rather than casein itself. Converted into solid casein, for instance by rennet, a ferment in the stomach, it is the basis of curds or cheese. When milk is drunk slowly, its casein content becomes a light and flaky mass of curds in the stomach, rather than an indigestible dense body. This action is significant for children, older persons, or invalids. Casein is not only high in nutritive values, but also has many industrial applications in the production of plastics, paints, and adhesives.

CASEIN – See article CARE AND FEEDING OF THE CHILD, page 1424.

CASTOR OIL, a pale yellow oil, expressed from the seeds of the ricinus or castor oil plant. It is an effective and prompt purgative and one of the oldest household remedies for constipation. It is likely, however, to be followed by costiveness and is therefore seldom used in chronic constipation. Castor oil is also used to counteract the effects of acid splashed in the eye.

The medicinal uses of castor oil have been recognized for centuries. It is mentioned in Egyptian papyri as an ideal purgative and as a stimulant for hair growth. The Incas of ancient Peru believed that castor oil possessed spiritual powers and used it to exorcise demons.

CASTOR OIL – See article THE FAMILY MEDICINE CHEST, pages 1250-51, 1254-55.

CASTRATION, the removal of one or both testes or ovaries, with a consequent deficiency of the endocrine hormones, testosterone and estrogen. It is one of the oldest surgical operations and was well known in earliest antiquity. Male foreign captives were castrated to prevent a mixing with foreign blood. Castration was sometimes a ritual which eliminated sexual desire so that an ascetic life could more easily be led. Among the self-imposed emasculates were Origen and St. Francis. At various times in history, especially in oriental countries, boys were castrated to become eunuchs. Later young male sopranos in church choirs were castrated so that their voices would not change. Castration as necessary medical surgery, too, was applied in cases of injury or disease. A castrated male was not always considered inferior; in fact, as in ancient Persia, he was sometimes highly esteemed and given important court positions.

Castration may be performed at almost any age. However, its effects are much more pronounced when performed before puberty. Removal of the testicles after puberty is accompanied by fewer symptoms because the body is fully developed. The early loss of testicular functions by injury, inflammation, or surgery results in definite characteristics. Castrated males, though often tall, are narrow-chested and effeminate, shy, gentle, placid, and lacking in endurance. Their voices are soft and highly pitched. While not necessarily bald, they do not have any hair on the face, armpits, and pubic areas. Obesity, especially layers of fat on the hips, are common, and pronounced breasts not unusual. Some of the secondary male sex characteristics do not change, however, if the operation is performed after the age of sixteen.

When the testicles are diseased or severely injured, castration is sometimes essential—for example, in cases of cancer of the prostate. Castration does not have any effect on sexual capacity, even though it has a pronounced one on sexual urge, and it does not prevent or increase susceptibility to mental breakdown. Castration must be differentiated from sterilization. Sterilization is not mutilating and does not interfere with sexual physiology; only the procreative capacity is eliminated.

Animals are usually castrated to make them plumper and more gentle, as well as to restrict capacity of reproduction. In females, castration, or spaying, consists in removing the ovaries, and is medically termed an oophorectomy.

CASTRATION – See article SEX HYGIENE, page 1667.

CASTRATION – cancer treatment: See article CANCER, pages 322-23, 347-48.

CASTRATION – hair growth: See article THE HAIR, page 945.

CATARACT, opacity producing loss of transparency of the lens of the eye; if the lens becomes entirely opaque, sight is lost. A cataract may be present at birth, and in young people it may appear as a result of injury. However, most cataracts occur in persons between the ages of fifty and seventy and are due to the gradual degeneration of the tissues of the lenses. To some extent, a tendency to this degeneration may be hereditary. Although the disease may show itself at first in only one eye, in almost all instances it will eventually appear in the other also. The process is gradual and "ripeness" or full opacity may take two years to develop.

Among the earliest symptoms of cataract are red eyelids, unexplainable daytime headaches, small specks seen constantly before the eyes, and gradually worsening vision. These or similar symptoms should be called promptly to the attention of a physician skilled in treatment of eye disorders. Temporary eyesight can be maintained by frequent changes of glasses.

Physicians generally agree, however, that the only effective treatment for a cataract itself is an operation. Such an operation restores good vision to approximately 97 persons out of a hundred. The surgery, relatively simple, is followed by the prescription of so-called cataract glasses, which contain biconvex lenses to replace the clouded natural lenses that are removed. *See also* EYE.

CATARACT – See article THE EYE, page 745-47.

CATARACT – diabetes: See article, DIABETES, pages 577-78, 587.

CATARRH, a term which was formerly used for inflammations of mucous membranes, especially those of the nose, throat, and the air passages. A cold with secretions—as a "running nose," for example—was popularly called a catarrh.

CATHARTICS, drugs or medicinal preparations that will relieve constipation and cause an evacuation of the bowels. Cathartics stimulate the muscular activity of the intestines and promote the flow of liquid to the bowels, thus flushing the alimentary canal. If the cathartic is especially strong, it is called a purgative. If it is mild, it is called a laxative.

Elimination of waste is a natural process, assisted by coarse foods, water, exercise, and laxative material in the diet such as fruit juices, vegetables, whole wheat, honey, and oatmeal. Most people can eliminate waste materials without artificial stimuli. The frequency of defecation—emptying the bowel—is not significant in most cases. If the use of cathartics appears to be frequently necessary a physician should be consulted. The habitual use of cathartics irritates the bowels, weakens their normal movement, and results in irregularity of elimination. The incidence of hemorrhoids, for example, is high among those who habitually use cathartics. In obesity, the prolonged use of cathartics is not only ineffectual but harmful.

Cathartics of any kind should never be taken when abdominal pain is present. This pain may be the first sign of a beginning appendicitis, and if an abdominal pain persists or appears to be exceedingly severe, medical treatment is imperative. When the appendix is inflamed, cathartics may increase the irritation and peritonitis may occur as a result. In many cases, such inflammation of the membrane which lines the interior of the abdominal cavity is fatal.

Mineral oil and mineral oil modi-fied with various substances are among the mildest of the cathartics currently used. Mineral oil is a lubricant which relieves constipation by mixing with the material in the bowel, softening it, and permitting easier passage along the intestinal tract. It is not fattening, as are other oils, because it is not absorbed by the bowels. The usual dose is one or two tablespoonfuls. Sometimes mineral oil is modified by the addition of agar, a form of seaweed, or by psyllium seed or other mucilaginous materials which swell when water is added and increase the bulk of waste material, thus preventing possible leakage of the oil from the anus, the excretory orifice of the body. However, too much mineral oil may interfere with the absorption of vitamin A. Mineral oil is also modified by the addition of strong laxative material like cascara and phenolphthalein. Cascara is a plant laxative made from the bark of a tree and is also available in the form of extracts and aromatic mixtures. Phenolphthalein is a laxative widely used as the basis of most advertised laxative remedies. This substance, which is a coal tar derivative, acts on the large intestine as a purgative. Some people are especially sensitive to phenolphthalein and in these cases its use will cause eruptions of the skin.

Other methods of relieving constipation are glycerin suppositories, enemas, and castor oil, an old household remedy. A tablespoon or two of milk of magnesia taken occasionally is considered a safe cathartic. Saline cathartics such as Epsom salt (magnesium sulfate), sodium sulfate, etc., are active cathartics, especially useful in inflammatory infections and as blood purifiers in cases of poisoning. *See also* CONSTIPATION; MEDICINE CHEST; and names of specific cathartics.

CATHETER, a flexible or rigid tube used to drain fluid from various cavities of the body, especially when the normal outlets do not function properly. The tube may be passed gently through the nose to the Eustachian tube which communicates with the ear, for example, or through the penis or vagina into the urethra which connects with the urinary bladder. A catheter should never be forced into or through any cavity.

Persons who use a catheter without professional assistance should remember that absolute cleanliness is essential. Before use, a catheter made of rubber or metal can be sterilized by being boiled in water for several minutes. If it is made of silk or some other material which could be damaged by boiling, it may be soaked in an antiseptic solution prescribed by the doctor. The hands of the person who passes the catheter should also be clean. When the catheter is to be passed through the urethra, the end of the penis or the outer surface of the vagina is ordinarily washed before the instrument is inserted. If difficulty is encountered in this process, an appropriate lubricant may be employed.

After use, the catheter should be thoroughly cleansed with soap and water. Grease may be removed with denatured alcohol. The catheter should be carefully dried and returned to a clean container. A worn catheter should be replaced.

CAUL AT BIRTH. Caul is a popular term for the sac in which the child lies during pregnancy. Part or all of this fetal membrane may be brought forth in labor, preceding the child. A caul at birth has sometimes been considered by superstitious people to be a sign of good luck.

CAUL AT BIRTH — superstitions concerning: See article CARE OF MOTHERS BEFORE AND AFTER CHILDBIRTH, page 1546.

CAUSALGIA, a sharp burning pain, sometimes a symptom of injuries of the nerves, particularly the sensory nerves supplying the palms and soles. The disturbance may be associated with many vasomotor, digestive, and dermal changes in the affected parts.

CAVITIES. See DENTAL CARIES.

CECUM, a portion of the bowel on the lower right side of the abdomen. It is the large blind pouch located at the junction of the large and small intestine. The appendix branches off the cecum.

CELIAC DISEASE, an ailment which affects children under five years of age, most frequently between the ages of two and three. In celiac disease, the child is unable to digest and utilize fats, starches, and sometimes sugars. Sensitivity to gluten from wheat or rye grains was recently established as the cause of this inability. The child becomes weak and undernourished, anemic, and his growth is stunted. Sometimes the stomach is swollen, as in starvation. Since the child is not well, he may be irritable, sullen, and behavior problems result as a consequence. Usually he has little appetite and even when obviously hungry will often refuse food. Conversely he may eat voraciously, with no gain in weight. Severe diarrhea is almost always the most telling symptom and stomach cramps may accompany it. Most of these symptoms are common to other conditions, and only a doctor can determine if celiac disease is the cause.

Celiac disease is ordinarily treated by a special diet. Fats, such as butter, cream, fried foods, and ice cream, and foods containing wheat or rye grains are excluded from the diet. Sugar tends to increase the amount of gas and to provoke diarrhea, and natural sugars, as are found in fresh fruits, are best tolerated. Protein foods can usually be eaten with no ill effect, and so milk protein, egg white, lean meat, fish, liver, and protein-rich vegetables constitute part of the diet. Of special benefit is a milk preparation which is high in protein but low in milk sugar and fat. For a time bananas were considered beneficial and banana diets were prescribed. However, now it is felt that any benefit derived from bananas is due to the fact that bananas replace gluten in the child's diet. Vitamin B complex supplements are also given.

CELL, a mass of protoplasm containing a nucleus; it constitutes the

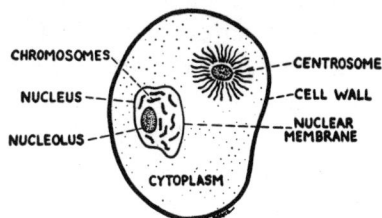

Cell—The unit of life. The single cell carries on all the processes necessary for maintaining life.

basic unit of life. *See also* BLOOD; BODY.

CELL – circulatory system supplies with essential materials and removes waste products: See article DISEASES OF THE HEART AND CIRCULATION, page 979.

CELL – growth: See article CANCER, page 319.

CELL – interstitial: See article SEX HYGIENE, page 1658.

CELL – mononuclear: See article INFECTIOUS DISEASES OF CHILDHOOD, page 1114-15.

CELL – red blood cells: See articles DISEASES OF THE HEART AND CIRCULATION, page 983-84; THE BLOOD AND ITS DISEASES, page 1025.

CELL – sperm: See article SEX HYGIENE, page 1658.

CELL – vaginal: See article THE KIDNEY: ITS DISEASES AND DISTURBANCES, page 1178.

CELL – white blood cells: See articles DISEASES OF THE HEART AND CIRCULATION, page 983-84; THE BLOOD AND ITS DISEASES, page 1025.

CELLULITIS usually refers to a diffuse inflammation of connective tissue. However, any inflammation of the cells of the body, at any point, can be called cellulitis. This disease may be caused by various bacilli, such as streptococci, staphylococci, or pneumococci.

CEREBRAL denotes anything that is related to the cerebrum, the chief portion of the brain. For example, the cerebral cortex, also called "gray matter," is the outer part of the cerebrum where most of the cell bodies are located. The cerebrum is divided by a deep groove into two cerebral hemispheres. These cerebral hemispheres are representative of approximately 70 per cent of the nervous system.

Illnesses associated with brain in-juries are denoted by the addition of the word "cerebral," as, for example, cerebral dysrhythmia which is epilepsy, and cerebral palsy or paralysis due to hemorrhage. *See also* BRAIN.

CEREBRAL ARTERIOSCLEROSIS. *See* SENILITY.

CEREBRAL HEMORRHAGE. *See* APOPLEXY.

CEREBROSPINAL MENINGITIS. Meningitis, as such, is not a definite disease but an inflammation of the meninges, the membranes of the brain and the spinal column. The invasion of the cerebrospinal column by microorganisms such as pneumococcus, staphylococcus, or streptococcus is usually responsible, but various viruses also cause meningitis.

Cerebrospinal meningitis, also called spotted fever and cerebrospinal fever, is a sporadic or epidemic form of meningitis caused by a germ, the meningococcus. This disease is characterized by inflammation of the cerebrospinal meninges.

While the cause of cerebrospinal meningitis is not yet fully established, medical scientists believe that it is spread by contact with germ-laden droplets, produced by coughing and sneezing, from the nose and throat of infected carriers. The incidence of the disease, which most frequently affects children and adolescents, is highest in winter and early spring. In its epidemic form, cerebrospinal meningitis sometimes occurs in overcrowded, unsanitary surroundings. Epidemics in schools are much less frequent than generally believed.

cervix are especially common after childbirth. Symptoms include profuse irritating discharge from the vagina and occasionally oozing of blood, especially after sexual relations. These infections may be treated with vaginal creams and suppositories, by painless treatment in the doctor's office, or with douches of prescribed medications. Sometimes a badly infected cervix may require surgery or cauterization. Cauterization involves burning away infected tissue with chemicals or electrical current.

Raw areas, erosions, may occur after delivery, and cause oozing of blood and irritating discharge. Their treatment is similar to that of infections. Treatments should be continued until the cervical infection or erosion is completely cured, for malignancy may develop in later years unless infections are entirely eradicated.

Fleshy warts which often grow on the cervix and sometimes cause bleeding are best removed by simple surgical measures. Cysts on the cervix may provoke bleeding or watery discharge. Treatment varies and is usually performed in the doctor's office.

Cancer can occur on the cervix and constitutes one of the most common types of cancer affecting women, especially after forty. Symptoms vary from none at all to bloody or irritating discharge. To verify his diagnosis, the doctor will take a small bit of suspicious tissue from the cervix for examination under the microscope. Should cancer be present, treatment includes complete surgical removal of all the internal female structures, and often the use of x-ray and radium. Only the doctor can decide which combination is best. Results in early cases are excellent. For this reason, all women over thirty-five years of age should have an internal examination every six months. *See also* CANCER.

CERVIX – See article CANCER, pages 321-22, 341-42.

CESARIAN SECTION, the surgical operation by which childbirth is accomplished when normal delivery is either dangerous or impossible. Each year, approximately 150,000 births occur in this manner, comprising 4 per cent of all deliveries. The operation was done in early times, and received its name from a law in the days of the Caesars stating that all pregnant women dying before giving birth be so delivered in hopes of saving the unborn child. Tradition has it that Julius Caesar was delivered this way, but this is refuted by the fact that Caesar's mother lived years after his birth.

Formerly, because of uncontrollable hemorrhage and infection, the operation was extremely hazardous, but today, in skilled hands, the risk is about the same as that in simple appendectomy. The technique of Cesarian section consists of entering by incision the abdomen and uterus in which the child develops during pregnancy. Once a woman has had one Cesarian section, future pregnancies are usually delivered by this operation, but occasionally normal delivery is possible. *See also* PREGNANCY AND PRENATAL CARE.

CESARIAN SECTION – See article SEX HY-

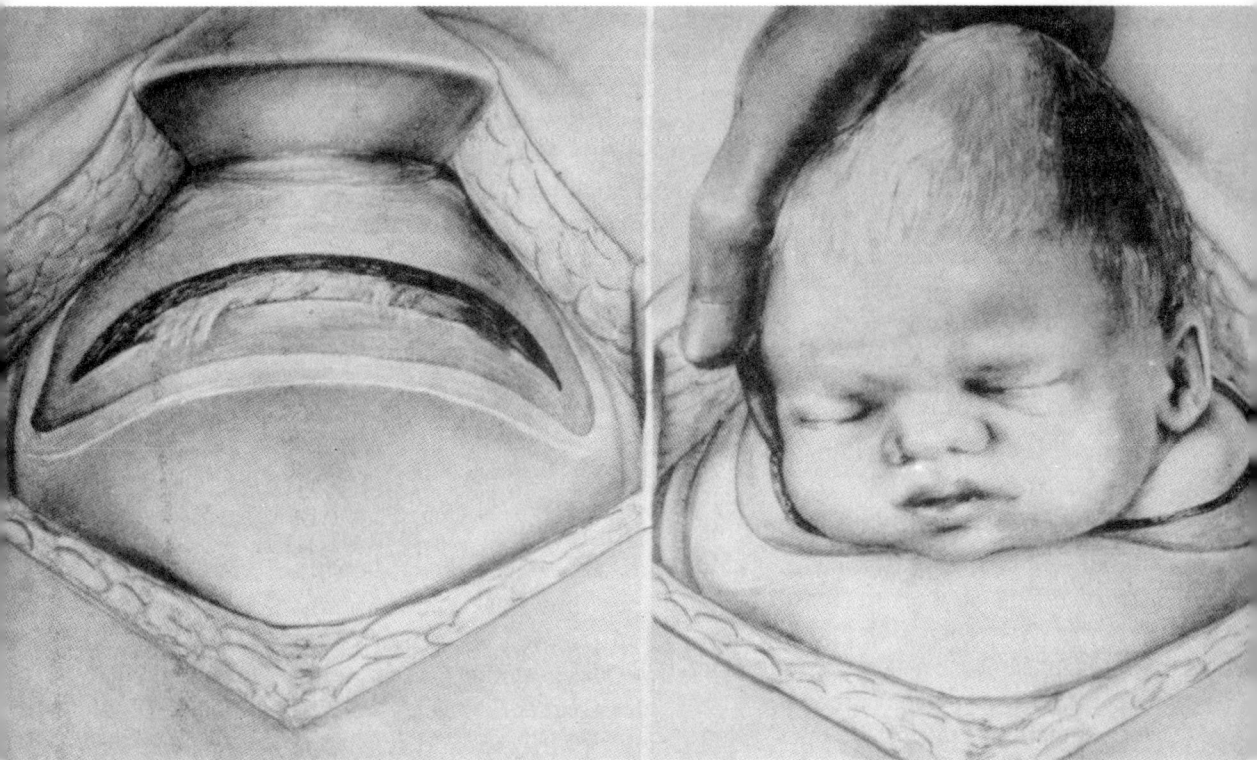

Cesarian Section — When the condition of the mother or size of the baby precludes delivery through the normal route, the physician does a cesarian section. A long slit is made in the abdominal wall and the uterus, which holds the baby, is opened *(left)*. The large object at the top of the drawing is a retractor holding back the flaps of skin. The baby is delivered through the opening made in the abdominal wall *(right)*. The surgeon holds the baby and carefully takes him out of the uterus. Cesarian section is done only when indicated because possibility of infection is high.

GIENE, pages 1689-90, 1704-05.
CESARIAN SECTION — superstitions: See article CARE OF MOTHERS BEFORE AND AFTER CHILDBIRTH, page 1544-45.

CHAFING, the irritation which results when two delicate skin surfaces persistently rub against each other, or when a foreign substance rubs the skin. The skin becomes red and painful and is often raw and moist. Chafing occurs most frequently under the armpits, in the groin, between the buttocks, below the breasts, in the folds of the skin, and also between the fingers and toes where it may be mistaken for a finger infection. Such an irritated area is a fertile place for germs or fungi.

For simple chafing, the treatment may consist of drying the skin thoroughly after bathing and applying a suitable dusting powder, zinc ointment, or cold cream, or one of the newer protective ointments. Cleanliness is important. Primarily essential, however, is the removal of the irritant which originally produced the lesion. This may mean more carefully fitted shoes, a larger, looser garment, or possibly a loss of weight. Sometimes a flat gauze bag filled with talcum powder and placed between the rubbing surfaces is soothing. *See also* ECZEMA.

CHAFING – See article THE SKIN, page 1748-50.

CHAFING – drugs to use: See article THE FAMILY MEDICINE CHEST, page 1254-55.

CHAGAS' DISEASE, (American trypanosomiasis), a tropical ailment found prominently in South and Central America. It is transferred to man by parasites, in the excretions of a blood-sucking bug which usually bites the human lips. In the human body these flagellate protozoans change into intracellular forms which infest the cells of the brain and heart, and therefore the symptoms of Chagas' disease resemble those of heart disease. Tissues are destroyed and the victim is incapacitated. A cure has not yet been found, and the fatality rate is high. Antibiotics have proved ineffective in Chagas' disease.

CHANCRE. The first visible symptom of syphilis is a sore, known as a chancre or hard chancre. The chancre usually develops from three to five weeks after exposure. It appears at the point where the spirochete has entered the body, which is ordinarily on the genital organs. Since it is possible, however, to contract syphilis without sexual contact, the chancre may occasionally appear in some other area, such as the mouth. If syphilis is treated in the primary, or chancre, stage, it can be cured with the use of antibiotics.

The term soft chancre, also known as chancroid, designates an inflammation of the genitals caused by an entirely different microorganism from that responsible for syphilis. The soft chancre, a yellow sore, discharging pus, appears a day or so after exposure. Unless the person is confined to his bed, so that his movements can be restricted to a minimum, the soft chancre may become an abscess. Swelling may also develop in the glands of the groin. Chancroid yields readily to treatment with proper hygiene and the use of antiseptics. Since syphilis may be involved, a physician should always be consulted. *See also* CHANCROID; SYPHILIS.

CHANCROID, a lesion in which the chancre, or sore, is soft, in contrast with the syphilitic chancre which is hard. It involves the genitalia and is usually of venereal origin. Chancroid was a fairly common disease in ancient Rome and is mentioned by several Roman historians. Early English writers sometimes referred to the disease, calling it the "groyne bump" or "Winchester goose," a name derived from the city of Winchester, where the disease was apparently widespread, and from the awkward gooselike walk of the victim.

The disease starts with an ache in the groin and inflamed glands. These swollen glands gradually gather into a painful poison-filled mass, called a bubo. Eventually the bubo bursts and the poison drains out. In many cases, the bubo remains open for weeks, and during this period the person may experience so much pain and discomfort that he is unable to walk.

Chancroid is a disease of uncleanliness, and is most common in dirty poverty-stricken areas where hygienic conditions are almost impossible to maintain. Its incidence is high in seaports and cities and towns with large transient populations.

Chancroid is caused by the streptobacillus of Ducrey and its incubation period is two to fourteen days after sexual intercourse. Treatment varies from washes and salves to caustics, electric cautery, and surgery. Sulfonamides are now an effective treatment, and antibiotics like streptomycin have also been successfully used.

CHAPPED SKIN, a roughened, reddened, irritable condition caused by loss of the natural oils in the skin. It occurs especially when the air is dry or when the skin is exposed to irritants such as cold hard water and harsh soap. Some persons are particularly susceptible to chapping because their skin glands do not respond to climate changes.

To prevent painful irritation of the skin, the use of soap and water during the winter months should be kept to a minimum. For personal use, mild oils may occasionally be used instead of soap and water, and fats in the skin replenished with cold creams, or lotions and creams, available in stores, which increase the moisture content of the skin. Rubber gloves or similar protective gloves may be used for household tasks.

The use of harsh soaps should be avoided. Hard water may be softened with washing soda or borax. A soft towel should be used to dry the hands; never a hot fire or an electric air drier. Lips, especially vulnerable to chapping because their sensitive surface is frequently moistened, may develop ugly painful breaks in the skin which are easily infected. A precautionary measure is to apply cold cream or petroleum jelly to the lips before going out into the cold. Chapped skin can be minimized if the home is properly heated, and overheat and excessive dryness avoided. A pan of water kept on the floor in each room will add moisture to the air through evaporation.

Despite all precautions, some chapping of the skin will occasionally occur. When this happens, the affected area should be protected from infection just as a wound is protected. Cracks in the skin may be treated with a mild ointment such as cold cream and then covered with clean gauze. If the irritation is prolonged, a physician should be consulted. *See also* CHILBLAINS; FROSTBITE; SKIN.

CHAPPED SKIN — See article THE SKIN, pages 1736, 1748-49.

CHEMOTHERAPY, the prevention or treatment of certain infectious diseases by various chemical agents which act as antiseptics in the body or inhibit invading parasites without producing serious toxic effects on the patient.

CHEMOTHERAPY — cancer research: See article CANCER, page 352-53.

CHEMOTHERAPY — cancer treatment: See article CANCER, page 322-23.

CHILBLAINS, an inflammation of the skin and of the tissues under the skin caused by cold; appears most often on the toes, fingers, ears, or nose.

The initial inflammation is followed by a burning or itching sensation, after which the area ordinarily becomes swollen and dark red. This color, as well as the characteristic chilled feeling, is due to a reduced circulation of blood in the area.

Those susceptible to chilblains should take protective measures. Warm clothing and carefully fitted warm shoes and gloves should always be worn during the winter months. Regular and vigorous exercise, such as walking and skating, is also advisable. Vulnerable areas of the body should be briskly massaged every day to encourage circulation of the blood. Regular doses of cod liver oil, as well as a healthful diet, are helpful, and general good health should be maintained.

Treatment of chilblains often includes painting the inflamed areas with a tincture of iodine. Zinc ointment is also beneficial. If blisters form, every effort should be exerted to prevent them from bursting, since healing is likely to be slow because of the condition of the affected area. If they do break, a stimulating ointment should be applied. A lotion composed of hydrogen peroxide and warm water in equal parts is useful for washing the sores, especially if they are discharging pus. *See also* FROSTBITE.

CHILBLAINS — See articles OCCUPATION AND HEALTH, page 1378-79; THE SKIN, page 1755-57.

CHILDBIRTH. *See* PREGNANCY AND PRENATAL CARE.

CHILD CARE

Many parents are bewildered by the responsibilities implied in the arrival of a new baby. They feel that they have before them a highly scientific task with which they, in their ignorance, will be unable to cope. This attitude is erroneous and should be discarded. There are facts about child care that should be

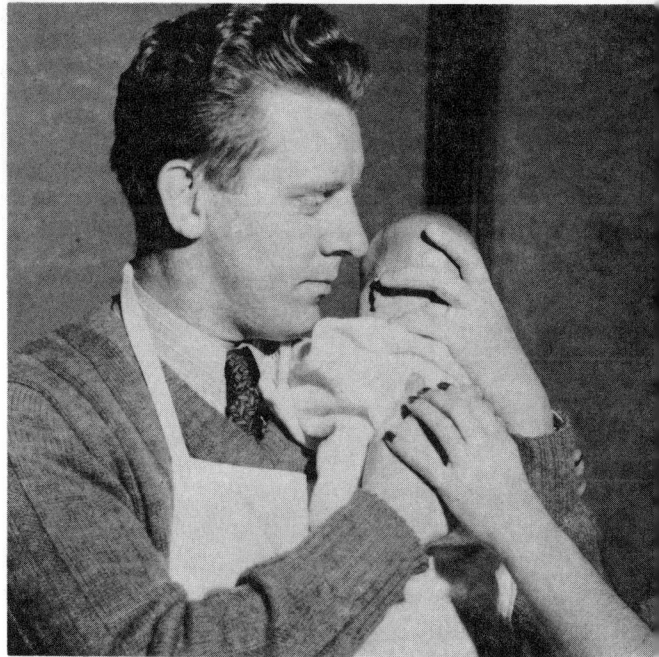

Child Care — Expectant fathers are interested in learning the correct ways to handle and care for the new baby. In special schools for expectant fathers instructions are received and techniques practiced until mastered. Photograph shows an expectant father as he practices the correct placement of hands and correct position of baby for "burping" after feeding. Dolls are used for demonstration purposes.

Three Lions, Inc.

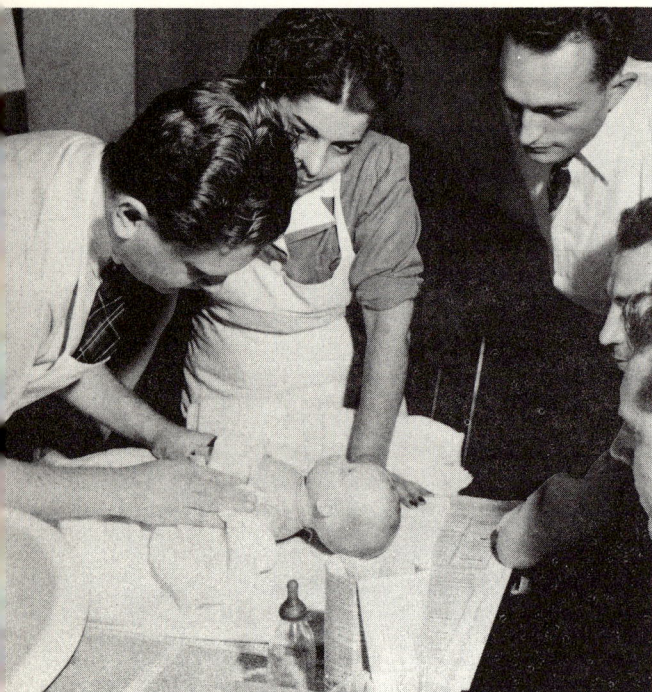

Child Care — An expectant father is learning how to bathe and dry the baby while other fathers-to-be look on. The doll is quieter than a live infant, but it provides good practice in handling tiny humans.
Three Lions, Inc.

known, but if parents use common sense and are really fond of their child they will not make serious mistakes.

In the 1920s, pediatricians had their information neatly packeted in concise crisp form and parents were told exactly what to do for their babies in each situation. More recently, however, pediatricians have discovered that babies cannot be treated in this rigid fashion. Just as babies are different from one another in size, hair color, eye color, and other characteristics, so are they different from one another in their likes and dislikes, in their feelings and

sleep habits, in their ways of growing, in their dispositions.

Babies should be treated as individuals; no one else can understand the idiosyncrasies of a baby as well as the parents. The parents should not expect the doctor to tell them what to do in every conceivable situation. He will guide and instruct the parents from his wealth of experience with babies in general, but they will have to apply what he tells them to their own baby. Parents must learn to rely on their own judgment not only because of the child's individuality but also because it is only through this hard schooling that they really acquire the art of parenthood. Theoretical knowledge and expert advice cannot take the place of practical experience.

Modern pediatrics has returned to a "naturalistic" attitude toward child care. The natural attitudes which grownups have assumed toward babies since the earliest days actually are the most desirable ones. It is good for the baby to be picked up from time to time, to be hugged and patted and rocked and sung to. Indeed, some pediatricians look to the time when the cradle will again have a place in the nursery.

Bringing up a baby should be a pleasure. If it is not, something is wrong with the situation. Parents will not enjoy their baby if they are worried because he is not getting enough vitamins or minerals, or because he has not been outdoors for several days, or because someone neglected to open a window in his room one night, or because he cried when a stranger approached, or because he weighs less than a neighbor's baby. Parents should learn to take it easy. If their baby is under a physician's care, they can rest assured that he is getting an adequate diet. Being indoors for a week or even longer will not hurt him; and, as for the weight of a neighbor's baby, it should be remembered that, within reasonable limits, there is no relation between health and happiness and body weight. Babies thrive best in a warm, affectionate, orderly atmosphere.

Structure and Growth. The average infant weighs about seven pounds at birth, girls generally weighing about half a pound less than boys, and Negro babies often weighing more than white. It is not unusual or abnormal for a child to weigh eight or even ten pounds. Babies born weighing less than five and a half pounds are classified as premature, regardless of how long the pregnancy has lasted, and require special care. Most babies will double their birth weight at six months of age and triple it at a year.

Length at birth is generally between nineteen and twenty-one inches and by the end of the first year the baby will have grown an additional ten inches. The baby's head and chest circumference should be equal at birth. Thereafter, the head size grows rapidly, increasing two and a half inches in circumference by the end of the first year. The bones of the skull are soft at birth

and often the skull is misshapen from the effect of labor and may be molded right after delivery. An odd-shaped head should not cause alarm; within a few weeks the skull will assume a normal contour. Since the bones of the baby's skull are soft and easily molded into an incorrect

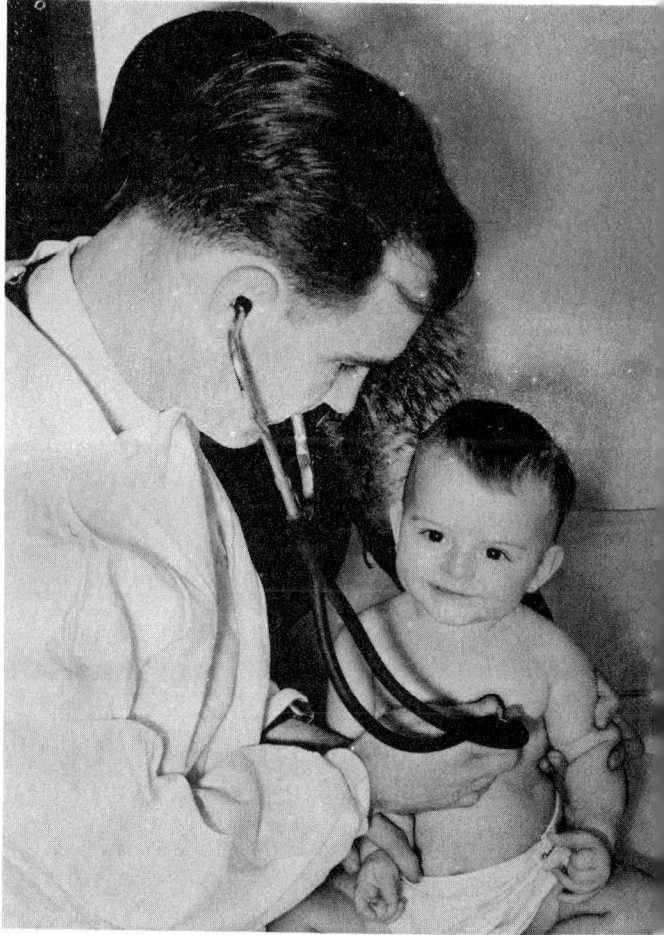

Child Care — Regular physical examinations are very important in the baby's life, especially during the first year. The baby grows so quickly that changes must be carefully watched. Regular check-ups are valuable because indications of poor health or faulty nutrition are detected early. Photograph shows a healthy, happy baby undergoing a complete examination.

shape, the infant should not lie in one position too long during the first year. He should lie on the left side after one feeding, on the right side after another, and be encouraged to sleep on both stomach and back. Fontanelles, the two soft spots in the skull, are places where the skull bones have not yet fused. The spot toward the back of the head usually fills in by the fourth month, and the spot in the front by the eighteenth month. Special care of the spots is not necessary, but they should not be disturbed.

PROGRESS CHART

One year

Weight: boys 21.5 pounds; girls 20 pounds

Height: boys 29.5 inches, girls 29 inches

Teeth: six by end of the year

Speech: Babbling; may say three to five words.

Two years

Weight: boys 28.4 pounds; girls 27.8 pounds

Height: boys 33.1 inches; girls 32.7 inches

Teeth: sixteen

Speech: vocabulary of 100 to 500 words; two-word sentences.

Three years

Weight: boys 33.5 pounds; girls 31.5 pounds

Height: boys 36 inches; girls 35.6 inches

Teeth: twenty

Speech: 500 to 1500 words; uses pronouns.

Four years

Weight: boys 36.4 pounds; girls 35.1 pounds

Height: boys 38.6 inches; girls 38.4 inches

Teeth: twenty milk teeth

Speech: makes complete sentences; 500 words added.

Five years

Weight: boys 41.4 pounds; girls 40.2 pounds

Height: boys 41.7 inches; girls 41.3 inches

Speech: articulation nearly perfect; shows an interest in rhyming.

Six years

Weight: boys 45.1 pounds; girls 43.6 pounds

Height: boys 44 inches; girls 43.4 inches

Teeth: twenty-four, four of which are permanent

Speech: articulation perfect; inflection of nouns and verbs almost perfect.

Learning to walk. Some children will begin to creep about the seventh month, while others sometimes wait until as late as the tenth or eleventh month. By the end of the first year the child should easily be able to pull himself into the standing position and to walk holding on to something. Usually he can walk at about eleven months if someone holds his hand. Walking unaided usually starts at about twelve to sixteen months. Of course, some children progress faster than others, but about 40 per cent of children can walk at a year, and 67 per cent at fourteen months.

Occasionally, if the child is fat or has been ill, he may not walk until the end of the second year. Sometimes a slippery floor or crowded play area, or ill-fitting shoes discourage the child from walking. Occasionally muscle disease, rickets, or nerve damage may be involved but this is rare. Parents should be patient with the child who is reluctant to start walking. Urging him to walk before he is ready can only make him insecure. Letting the child play with other toddlers will encourage him to imitate them and try to walk himself.

Seeing and Hearing. At birth, babies can distinguish between light and dark, but they are not able to fix their attention on any object until about two weeks of age when the eyes can focus on light. Usually, at four weeks, the child can look at something and at two months follow a moving object with his eyes. During the first few months, difficulty in focusing correctly the delicate eye muscles may cause the eyes to look crossed. Parents should not be alarmed since this difficulty normally disappears soon.

Babies recognize noises and voices soon after birth, but are unable to distinguish specific sounds for two or three months. An infant of two or three months enjoys listening to music and often will stop crying if the radio or phonograph is turned on softly.

Babies do not have a developed sense of taste as a rule and can usually distinguish only between sweet and sour foods.

The first six years. The most rapid growth period in a child's life is the first four months. At one month, the baby will look at a person near by,

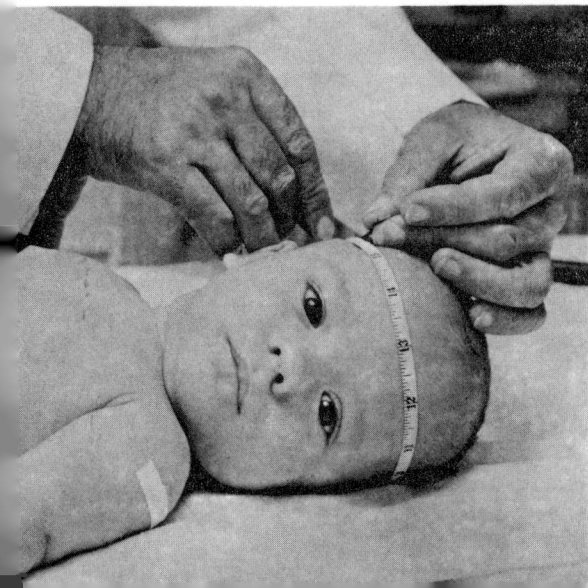

Child Care — The mental alertness and awareness of the baby can be measured. Photograph shows a cube being held forward to test the prehensile and interest attitudes of the child. The baby's mental development as well as physical growth should be checked at frequent intervals.
Three Lions, Inc.

Child Care — The head grows rapidly during the baby's first year of life. The cranial measurements are being taken as a part of an extremely careful and thorough check-up.
Three Lions, Inc.

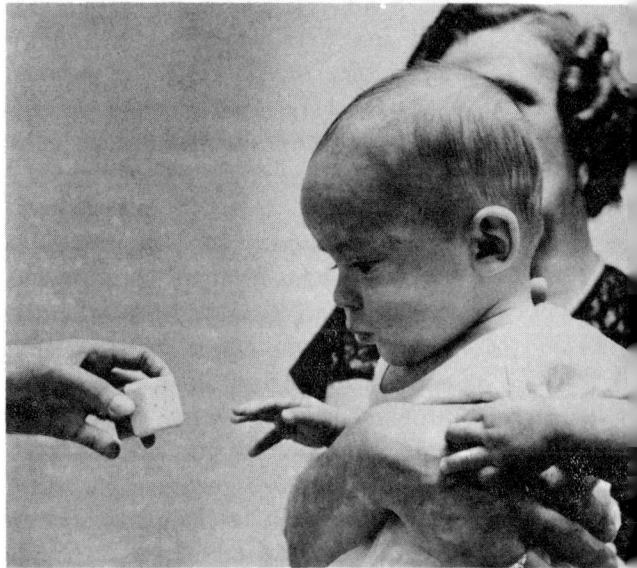

hold objects placed in his hand. His eyes can follow a moving object and he can hold his chin up when lying on his stomach. Whether or not the child really smiles, or just has a gas bubble in his stomach, is difficult to say, but at two months he definitely smiles when he sees his parents and persons who give him attention or when he feels contented. The two-month-old baby will coo, hold up his chest when prone, and turn his head away from bright lights. He turns toward a spoken voice and sometimes is frightened by loud noises.

At three months the baby can hold his head steady and may laugh. He can roll over, so it is not safe to leave him unprotected on an open bed. He gurgles and grasps objects. He may prefer his mother or whoever takes care of him to anyone else.

A four-month-old baby loves to study his hands, fingers, and objects around him. His attention is easily distracted by the world around him and feeding time may become a problem.

By five months, the child will sit propped, and recognize and be afraid of strangers. He will begin to scratch and to put toys in his mouth.

By the end of the sixth month, the child may sit briefly without support, reach for things he wants, and pound on furniture. He will probably love to watch himself in the mirror, and will stretch his arms to go to his parents or those he likes.

When he is seven to eight months, the baby will play peek-a-boo, pick up small objects, and often stand, if

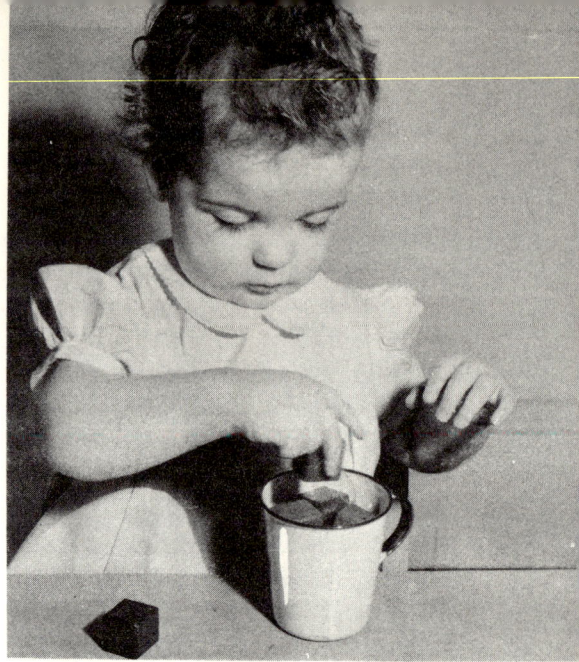

Mental Growth — What a child does with blocks is a good test of mental growth. Though monotonous to the adult observer, this girl's activities are everything one could desire of a child her age. Given a cup and a set of blocks, she will continue filling and emptying the cup endlessly until distracted.
Three Lions, Inc.

held. He may pull his mother's hair, and can wave good-bye.

In the last four months of the first year, the child will begin to recognize his own name and names of persons around him. He can open boxes, play with appropriate toys, walk alone or by holding on, notice other babies, and repeat simple words.

Speech is a significant means of testing development of the child. At the age of one year, a child can say a few simple words.

Dr. Arnold Gesell, child psychologist, states that at two years of age the child should be able to fold paper, name familiar objects such as keys, pennies, and watches, listen to stories, look at pictures, and attempt to describe his own experiences. He will ask for things by their own names and begin to make sentences of about two to three words.

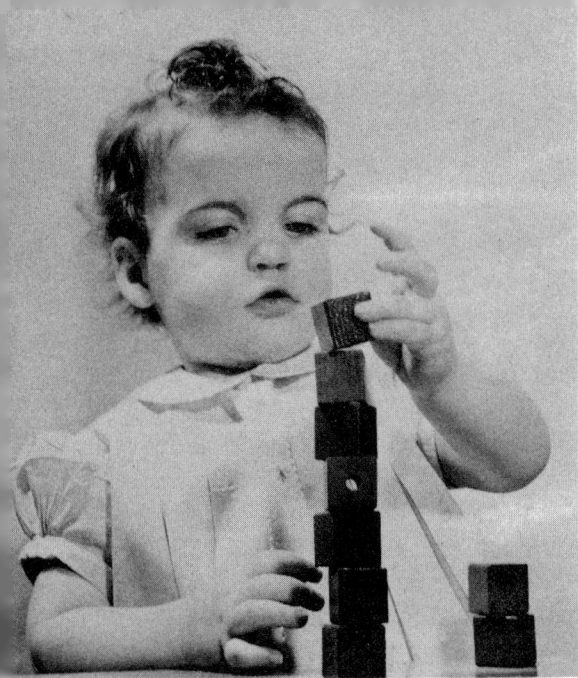

Mental Growth — Photograph illustrates the mental development of this child. Given a number of blocks, she will begin to pile them one on top of the other without further direction. She will not, at this age, build in two directions, but will continue piling them only in a vertical column.

Three Lions, Inc.

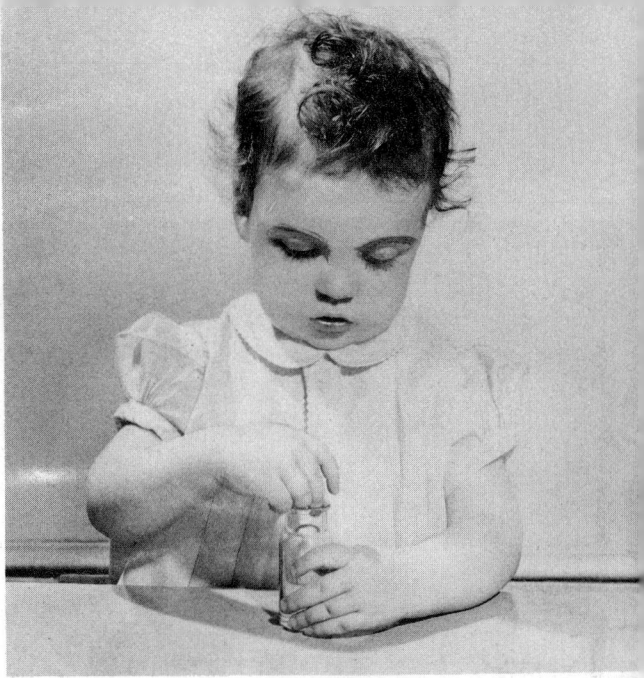

Mental Growth — Testing the baby's mental development. Fine motor movements permit precise grasp of the small pellet given this child. She is able to drop it into the flask without any trouble. Given two objects such as these, most any child of this age will proceed to use them in this way.

Three Lions, Inc.

According to the Stanford-Binet tests, at three years of age the child of average intelligence will be able to point out his mouth, nose, and eyes and repeat two numbers, but not consecutively. He will look at a picture and pick out four or five objects meaningful to him such as a boy, dog, tree, or car. Most children do these things quite easily, and failure to accomplish these simple tests may necessitate special training.

At four, the child should know his sex, and be able to name three familiar objects shown to him, such as a spoon, book, and pencil, and to repeat three nonconsecutive numbers.

At six, the child should know whether it is noon or evening, and to define the use of a fork, chair, knife, or table.

Crying. Physiologists recognize the value of crying for the new baby. Crying helps ventilate the baby's lungs, forcing out old air and replacing it with fresh air. The thrashing about of arms and legs associated with crying helps develop the body musculature. Also crying is the only way a baby can indicate his needs, whether it be food, sleep, a change of diapers or love, to those around him.

Most of the time a baby cries because he is uncomfortable, and parents should check for wet or soiled diapers or an open safety pin. The child may be too hot or cold. Often crying may indicate fear or anger. A new baby enjoys being in command and if he learns that he can control adults by crying he will continue to do so. Always be sure when the baby cries that he is comfortable, dry, and has had enough to eat.

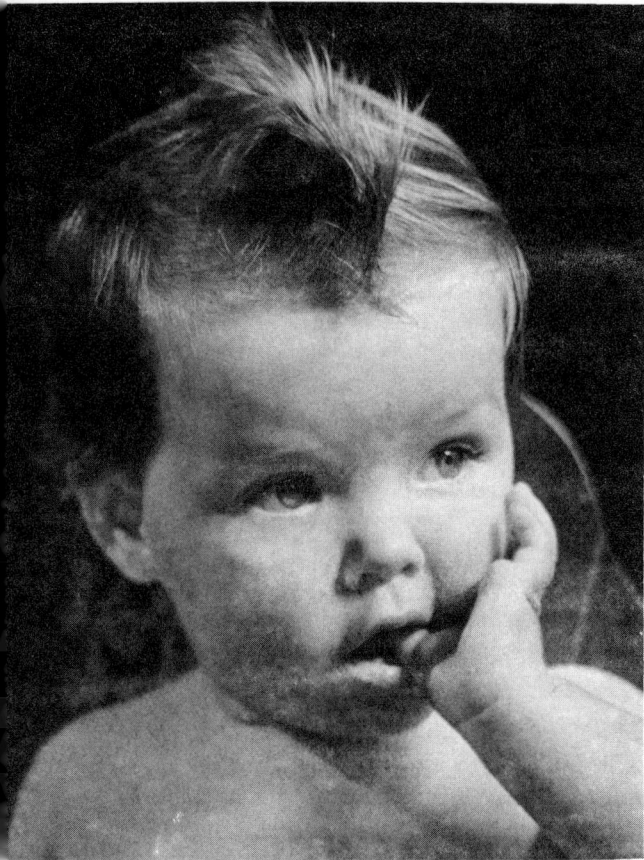

Thumb-sucking—Thumb or finger sucking can cause malocclusion which may result in facial disfigurement. To prevent irregular growth of teeth this habit should be stopped early.

Thumb sucking. Practically all babies, some more than others, suck their thumbs. In moderation, thumb sucking does not do any harm and interference with the eruption of teeth will ordinarily not happen unless the habit continues past two years of age. Thumb sucking may indicate that the child is hungry or unhappy. It frequently occurs among babies who are weaned too soon, thus depriving them of the pleasurable satisfying practice of sucking.

Artificial devices to prevent thumb sucking, such as arm splints or bitter preparations on the thumb, should not be used. It is better to try to find out the reason why the baby sucks his thumb. He may need more love and security. His hand should not be pulled out of his mouth, and the parents should avoid appearing upset about the habit. Ordinarily the child will discontinue sucking his thumb before the habit is prolonged enough to harm him.

Bed wetting. Children usually learn bladder control during the daytime some time during the end of the second year. Nighttime control may not occur until the third or even fourth year, but ordinarily it is accomplished by the end of the third year. If persistent bed wetting continues beyond four years of age, consult the doctor.

Bed wetting may arise from emotional reasons, such as insecurity or jealousy of a new baby in the family. It can also occur if parents are too vigorous and rigid in insisting on

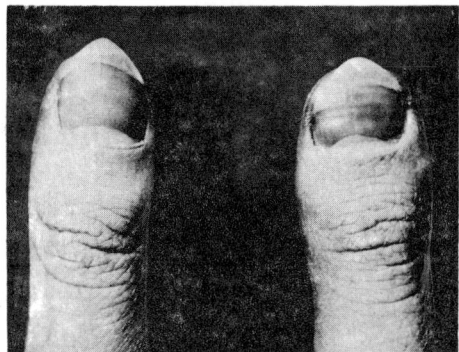

Thumb-sucking—If the bones are soft and the habit persistent, the thumb may be deformed by thumb-sucking. Photograph shows the difference in formation of thumbs in a patient who had the thumb-sucking habit during childhood.

384

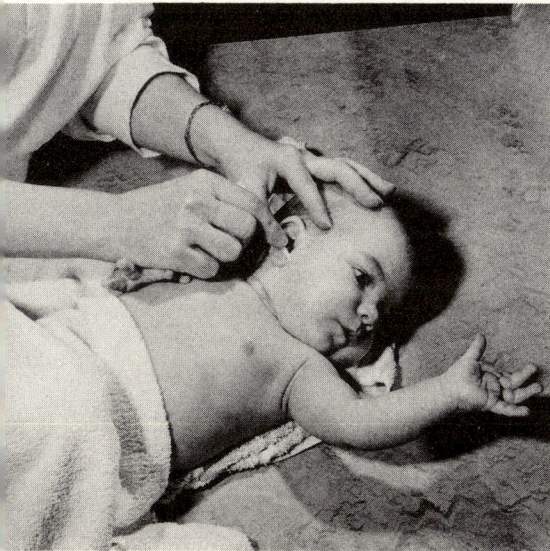

Ear, Nose and Throat — The baby undergoes a thorough ear, nose and throat examination. Note that the doctor and nurse wear masks to prevent spreading germs. Young babies are very susceptible to infections.
Three Lions, Inc.

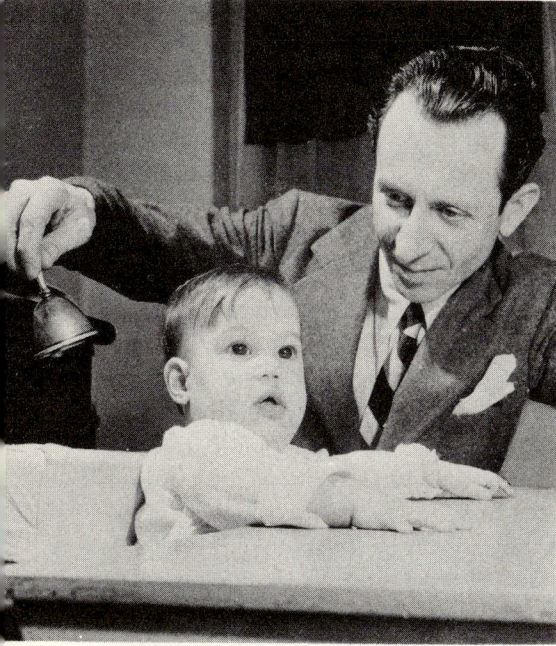

Hearing — A physician is testing the baby's response to a ringing sound. As unresponsive as they sometimes seem, babies are nevertheless capable of showing a great variety of responses indicative of their ability to comprehend simple situations.
Three Lions, Inc.

Ear — The baby's ears should be cleaned regularly. Photograph shows the correct technique for this operation. The movements should be gentle and the swab is never inserted deep into the canal.
Three Lions, Inc.

Nose and Throat — The physician examines the baby's nose and throat carefully on every office visit. Babies are especially susceptible to respiratory infections. Every precaution should be taken to keep the baby from catching cold.
Three Lions, Inc.

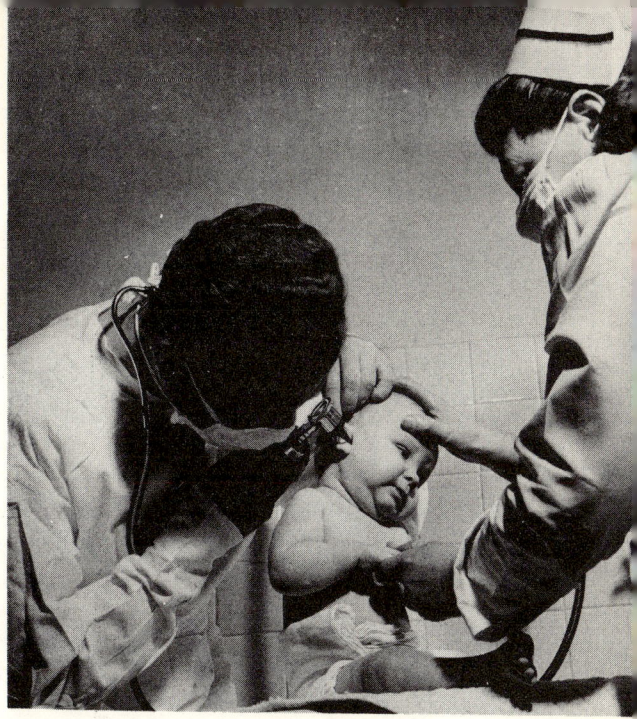

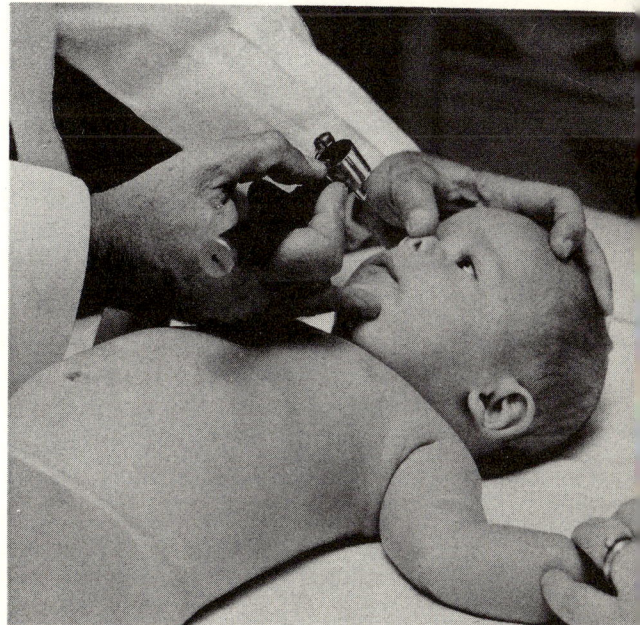

All mothers should make every effort to breast feed their babies, since breast-fed infants have a much lower incidence of infection, and seem to develop a little faster. In only rare instances does the milk of the mother fail to agree with the child. Occasionally diarrhea occurs if some element in the mother's diet disagrees with the child, but this can easily be detected and corrected in most cases.

Diet for nursing mothers. A common belief persists that a mother who wants to produce sufficient good rich milk for her baby should eat plentifully, drink excessive amounts of milk, cocoa, or even beer. This is not true; many women who have done this have become unpleasantly fat, disgusted with nursing, and inclined to discontinue. Actually the diet for a nursing mother is little different from that of any healthy adult woman, with about an extra quart of fluid, half of which is whole milk, each day. The diet should be about 2500 to 3000 calories, which usually does not lead to any increase in the mother's weight. The nursing mother should avoid taking substances such as strong laxatives which deplete her body's fluid resources, or stimulate the kidneys, such as excessive amounts of coffee or tea.

The theory that a nursing mother should avoid gassy or sour foods such as cabbage, salads, and raw fruits is also without foundation, unless, of course, she herself is allergic to a particular food. Fried foods may be eaten when a woman is nursing, but it is best to avoid chocolate since many people are sensitive to it. The best flow of milk results from regular nursing of the baby because the sucking action actually stimulates the formation of milk in the mother.

The diet of the nursing mother should contain about one quart of milk each day, some butter, four eggs a week, two green vegetables daily, and fresh fruit every morning, particularly oranges or tomatoes which are rich in vitamin C. Butter provides vitamins A and D; to provide a full supply of these vitamins the mother may take cod liver oil as directed by her doctor. The milk drunk daily may be whole, or nonfat dry milk if she is overweight. If she doesn't wish to drink milk, it may be used in food such as ice cream, custards, or cocoa drinks.

Mothers often worry about taking medicine, fearing that it will appear in the breast milk and harm the baby. Actually few drugs will do this, but if in doubt consult the doctor.

Secretion of milk begins a few days after the baby is born. In some cases, the breasts may leak fluid during the last few weeks of pregnancy. During the first few days, the flow is usually scanty but becomes more profuse by the end of the first week if nursing is frequent and the child is hungry enough so that he sucks vigorously. The first secretion of milk is actually not milk, but a cheesy protein-rich substance known as colostrum which appears about the third day and is nourishing for the baby. Later the true milk begins and is pale bluish white in color, resembling skim milk. This color is normal and does not mean that the milk is weak.

By the end of the first week, the average mother should have no difficulty secreting a pint of milk daily. This gradually increases and by the sixth month she is producing a quart of milk daily. The amount produced usually parallels the demands of the baby. Complete emptying of the breasts at nursing time is desirable to encourage good milk production. Nursing from both breasts at each feeding is recommended until maximum production is established. Then alternate the breasts to avoid overproduction.

Mature milk which is secreted by the mother after the first month is about 87.5 per cent water, 1.25 per cent protein, 7.5 per cent sugar, and 3.5 per cent fat. Breast milk is considerably sweeter than cow's milk, though somewhat lower in protein. It is also much more digestible and breast-fed babies are less apt to regurgitate or have gastrointestinal upsets. Through the mother's milk they also receive protective antibodies against disease which are not found in cow's milk. If the mother's diet is insufficient, the milk will be poor in quality. Vitamins should be taken by the nursing mother to enrich the milk.

Smoking does not affect the milk, and alcohol may be taken in moderation while the mother is nursing since it does not pass into the milk except in small amounts.

Hygiene during nursing. The nursing mother should keep in good physical condition and eat properly, and allow for a good night's sleep with a rest period in the midafternoon and, if possible, before nursing

periods. Worry and overfatigue are to be avoided.

The size of the breasts does not seem to be linked to supply of milk and women with smaller breasts often produce the most milk. Determining in advance whether or not a mother will be able to nurse her baby is not possible. Certain women should not nurse, however. These include those women who are not in good health, those who have active tuberculosis or other infections, those who have had arduous labors, and those who have previously had tumors of the breast or breast infection. If the breasts become infected while nursing, it should be discontinued. Premature babies thrive on mother's milk, but often their sucking power does not permit nursing. In some hospitals the mother's milk is drawn off by a breast pump and then fed to the baby with an eye dropper or small tube until it is strong enough to nurse by itself.

If the baby begins vomiting or fails to gain weight, the mother probably should stop nursing. However, she should consult the doctor first. Failure to nurse one child need not imply that future attempts will be unsuccessful.

Frequency of feeding. Babies are usually given their first feeding about twelve to twenty-four hours after birth. The feeding is started at about four-hour intervals. If the mother does not have milk, sugar-and-water solutions may be fed to the baby.

Although opinion as to how often to feed the baby varies, most doctors seem to favor a three- or four-hour schedule. During the first few days it may be necessary to nurse the baby more often but the interval should not be less than two hours. In short time, most babies seem to wish to be fed every four hours and by the sixth week sleep through the night and do not wake up to be fed. Babies should never be awakened just to feed them unless their sleep pattern becomes set in such a way that the entire household is upset. One theory favors letting the baby get hungry before feeding him, since usually he will not only nurse more vigorously but also take more at each feeding. Generally, after being fed, the baby will sleep for several hours. When he awakens he may be wet or need to expel gas and cry, which does not necessarily mean that he has not received enough to eat.

Nursing should take place in a quiet surrounding. The mother should lie down on her bed or sit in another comfortable position during the feeding. Prolonged nursing is not desirable and may lead to irritation of the nipples and not more than ten or fifteen minutes should be allowed for nursing. Studies show that the food obtained after the first six to eight minutes is hardly sufficient to be significant. Breast-fed babies develop strong sucking powers and can empty the breast rapidly. Mothers should be sure to "burp" the baby about halfway through the feeding. Once the baby is on a regular feeding schedule, it is desirable to try to maintain it, except in unusual cases.

Overfeeding and underfeeding. If the baby seems fretful after nursing and does not rest or sleep, the mother's milk may be insufficient. In such cases, the doctor will prescribe a supplementary formula to be given after the regular nursing period.

Most babies stop nursing when they have had enough and seldom does a nursing baby overfeed. Occasionally, however, a baby getting too much milk too fast may vomit or regurgitate, or have an upset stomach afterward, but this is rare. If it does occur, the nursing time should be shortened.

It is not advisable to weigh the baby before and after the feeding to see how much milk he gets; this is not only bothersome but may also disturb the mother unnecessarily. The behavior of the baby after the feeding is the best indication of whether or not he has received the proper amount. After nursing, hold the baby for a few minutes until he is ready to sleep. If he sleeps satisfactorily for two or three hours, he has had enough to eat.

Cow's milk. Generally the formula for babies is based on cow's milk, which should be pasteurized to remove harmful bacteria and purchased from a reliable dairy or market. In country homes where milk is obtained directly from cows, the milk must be boiled immediately after being drawn, then strained through cheesecloth into thoroughly boiled and sterilized bottles, cooled promptly, and placed in the refrigerator. In cities, these precautions are not necessary since milk is produced and pasteurized under the supervision of a health department. Heating milk does not remove any nutritional factors but does kill bacteria which may cause infections with streptococci or transmit tuberculosis, typhoid, diphtheria, or scarlet fever. Heating also helps to increase the digestibility of cow's milk. Because the vitamin C in the milk, essential to the child, may be destroyed by heating, it is customary to begin giving the child diluted orange juice or vitamin drops at two weeks of age.

Directions for feeding a baby with cow's milk should be obtained from the doctor. Cow's milk varies in composition from human milk, but in the formula must simulate breast milk. Ordinarily the baby cannot digest plain cow's milk until he is six months old and should receive it only upon suggestion and supervision of the doctor.

Preparing the baby's formula. When preparing the formula, all equipment needed should be washed thoroughly and boiled daily. The top of the bottle or can containing the milk must be washed with hot water and soap and rinsed thoroughly. Mix and measure the ingredients in sterilized containers, wash and boil the bottles to contain the formula, and close with sterilized rubber nipples. Individual bottles for each feeding are preferable to one large bottle from which the milk is measured. To provide for accidents, such as breakage or contamination, make one extra bottle. It is usually easier to make the whole day's supply in advance, preferably in the morning. After the feedings are prepared, the formula should be placed in the re-

frigerator. Nipples should be made of thin rubber, washed and boiled daily, and rinsed after use to extend their life.

Before feeding the baby, the mother should wash her hands well with soap and water. The bottle can be warmed by placing it in a pan of water on the stove. To test the temperature, shake a drop or two of the formula on the inside of the wrist. It is best to let a spray of milk run out until the drops fall one by one. In some cases, the holes in the nipple may need to be enlarged, which can be done by heating a pin over a flame and plunging it into the top of the nipple.

Cleanliness in the care of the baby's feedings is essential when he is young to protect him against serious infection. Sterilization is not essential after six to nine months, but the equipment should continue to be carefully cleaned before use.

Changes in the formula should be made only on the advice of the doctor because the baby's stomach and digestive system are extremely sensitive. If the baby seems healthy and continues to gain weight, there is ordinarily no need to change the formula. If he fails to gain weight, or if diarrhea or constipation occurs, the doctor may prescribe a new formula with an increase or decrease or adding or elimination of some ingredient.

A baby's weight gain is not always continuous. If he drinks greedily and rapidly, cries for more, or gets fretful long before feeding time, he probably needs more food. But the baby may be crying for other reasons and the mother should be sure that underfeeding is the reason before increasing his food, or overweight may occur. At one time, fat babies were considered the healthiest babies but this idea has been disproved and in fact the opposite may be true. The baby should never be deliberately overfed. He can handle so much food a day and beyond his limit will become upset and nauseated.

Water requirements. In relation to his weight, an infant needs about three times more water than an adult. His output of heat is greater and his body metabolism requires more water. Therefore, he occasionally ought to receive a bottle of lukewarm water. In winter, especially in dry apartments, he may awake fretful, with a dry throat, and need a few swallows of water to quench his thirst. The total fluid intake, including milk, water, and juice, of a growing baby should be about three ounces per pound of his weight, and a little more in hot or dry climates.

Feeding with spoon and cup. Food or a few drops of juice or formula on a spoon may be given to the infant when he is just a few weeks old. This will prepare him to use a spoon for solids later. At first he may appear to spit out the food because he cannot control his tongue. To prepare the baby for drinking from a cup, let him sip his daily orange juice from a small glass. Some babies do this easily, others find it difficult. By the sixth to ninth month, many babies can drink successfully from a cup. If, during the first few attempts, the baby shows any reluctance to drink from a cup, further attempts should be discontinued for a few weeks. Even if he cannot drink from a cup by one year, the parents should not be alarmed. He will learn to do this by imitating those around him, and forcing will only disturb him.

Solid foods. At the end of the first month, most babies can begin to take solid foods mixed with formula or water. The baby may begin with bran, rice, or oat cereal; avoid cereals containing wheat until he is nine months old. The foods should be given in small amounts, thinned with formula or water so that the baby can swallow them more easily. After the cereals are well established in his diet, vegetables are tried one by one, carrots, peas and string beans first. It is usually cheaper and more convenient to purchase the vegetables already cooked and strained and ready to eat after a slight warming. At three months, the baby can begin to eat fruit; at four to five months, meat. When the baby is seven or eight months old, if he has teeth, he may begin on the junior foods, which are coarser and must be chewed slightly. They should not be given until the baby's teeth appear and he is able to eat the food without fuss. A new food should be introduced in a small amount, only a teaspoonful, and then increased according to the baby's appetite. A boiled potato may be given when the child is seven months old; crackers, zwieback, dried bread or toast added when the teeth appear. Substances eaten by the baby may appear in the bowel movements, and this should not cause alarm. By ten or eleven months, the baby may eat many of the easily digested foods that the rest of the family are served, if they are cut up or chopped.

Schedule for the one-year-old child. When the child is a year old, he will be eating approximately as follows.

Upon arising, he should have from 7 to 8 ounces of milk. About 8:30 he receives breakfast of cereal, fruit and, if the doctor recommends it, egg yolk.

At noon, the baby should have 4 to 6 ounces of vegetable or meat broth, or one egg, or as a third possibility some scraped or chopped meat. To this may be added some white vegetables, such as 2 tablespoons of potato or rice, and from 2 to 4 tablespoons of a green vegetable, such as string beans, peas, or spinach. He may also drink more milk.

In the evening, around six, he should have cereal and milk, and also a cracker or small piece of toast, and 1 or 2 tablespoons of cooked fruit, which has a slight laxative quality.

Babies thrive best on a strict daily schedule. Occasionally exceptions must and should be made in his daily routine, but they should be kept to a minimum.

Self-feeding. At the end of the first year, babies ordinarily show an interest in self-feeding and can pick up pieces of carrot, potato, or toast. Actual self-feeding should be accomplished by the end of the second year. Rarely is there need to feed a child after this time. The child should eat a variety of foods at mealtime, and the mother see to it that the diet is well-balanced and the food attractively prepared. The child should drink water several times between meals, but soft drinks and candies should be avoided.

Most pediatricians recommend that food be given at regular intervals, and removed if not eaten in a reasonable time, about twenty minutes, and the child not given more food until the next regular meal. Coaxing the child to eat does little good and should be avoided.

Cleanliness. The child should have a complete bath at least twice a week after the first year and preferably one every day, before bedtime. Washing the hands should be encouraged during the second year. The child, if he plays as he should, is likely to get dirty and disheveled. The mother should not badger the child to remain clean, although it is wise if the mother teaches the child to clean up following play and meals.

The young child's hair should be shampooed about every three or four days, according to the season, and oils need not be used afterward.

Cleanliness will become more habitual if it is made easy—the soap and washstand within easy reach, the mirror low enough for the child to see himself, and the towel readily available. This does not mean that child-size bathrooms are necessary, but perhaps it might require a steady firm stool or box on which the child can stand. It helps the child if one of his parents washes or brushes his teeth at the same time as the child, since children love to imitate and learn best this way.

Feeding the older child. At one year of age, the child will probably be able to eat some of the foods that the family is eating, unless he has an allergy to one of them or does not have enough teeth to chew his food well. Eggs should be taken easily in all forms by one year. While egg yolk is started at six months, egg white should not be given until the end of the first year.

Cod liver oil. In the United States, cod liver oil or vitamin compounds in liquid form are practically universally given to children daily. Cod liver oil contains large amounts of vitamins A and D, which prevent or help cure rickets. In rickets, softening of the bones occurs due to failure of the body to use properly the mineral substances calcium and phosphorus. Vitamin D is the essential material involved in utilization of these minerals and so should be added to the diet in plain or mint-flavored cod liver oil, or through other vitamin preparations. Vitamin D is created by the body from exposure to sunshine in the summer, so most children do not need supplements at that time; but they are essential in the winter. At one time 50 to 80 per cent of children developed rickets; their bones did not grow properly and their muscles were flabby. Now milk is often fortified with vitamin D and additional vitamins are also given. Cod liver oil in straight form is also prescribed by some doctors.

Sleep for the baby. Newborn babies with good digestion and good appetite, plus proper foods, will usually sleep about nine-tenths of the time. Gradually they require less sleep, so that by the age of six months they sleep only about fifteen hours a day; from then until they are six, about twelve hours; from seven to ten years, eleven hours a day; from eleven to fourteen years, ten hours a day. Nine hours of sleep are needed by older teen-agers. Up to six years, a child should also have a nap during the day, lasting from 45 minutes to an hour and a half.

A baby should sleep in a room that is darkened and away from routine household noises. Hunger, pain, sudden noises, flashes of light, and sudden changes in temperature will awaken a small baby. The child will sleep soundly if he is warm, but not overly warm, well fed, and in a quiet darkened room. A baby often tends to wake up at a slight sound, and so the mother should not rush into his room every time he whimpers, even at night.

A baby should be put to bed at a reasonably early hour, usually around six o'clock, and not kept up late, unless for a good reason. Frequently an overtired child has difficulty going to sleep and will be cranky and irritable the following day.

The mattress on which a baby sleeps should be firm, but soft enough to be comfortable. The child should be lightly covered and his room comfortably warm, but not hot. In good weather, the window may be open enough to permit fresh air to circulate freely. Pillows are not necessary until the third year.

In nice weather, naps may be

taken out-of-doors as early as two weeks of age; in winter, not until six weeks. If it is inconvenient to put the baby outside, he can be placed in his carriage next to an open window, with the door of the room shut to avoid draft. In cold weather, cold cream applied to the baby's face will protect its delicate skin.

Clothing. Most mothers dress the baby too warmly, and as a result the child perspires excessively and may kick off his covers and then become chilled. There has been much discussion whether or not a baby should wear cotton, wool, silk, rayon, or mixtures of these fabrics. Cotton is usually not warm, since it carries off heat rapidly. However, it can be easily boiled or sterilized and is useful for diapers and summer clothes.

Because it conducts heat poorly, wool is a warm material, but it is somewhat irritating to the skin and is often difficult to launder. Wool must be washed with lukewarm water and mild soap since boiling or hot water and strong soap harden and otherwise harm its fibers.

Silk is not a warm material and some babies are sensitive to it. Rayon, too, is not particularly warm and must be washed with some care.

Sleeping bags. The sleeping bag is very useful for the baby. Correctly sized and constructed, it is loose enough to permit plenty of motion and warm enough to prevent loss of heat. Also, it cannot be kicked off during sleep. Care must be taken that the sleeping bag fits loosely, particularly around the wrists and neck, and that it is long enough to permit the baby to stretch. Materials used

may be sheeting, canton flannel, French flannel, or light blanketing, the choice depending upon the season.

Protective pants. Protective pants, made of various materials such as rubber, plastic, and rubberized silk, are a great convenience. To avoid skin irritation, they should be replaced by dry ones when the baby's diaper is changed. Washing immediately prolongs the life of the pants. If the child has irritated buttocks, avoid continuous use of the pants. They should fit loosely around the legs and waist. The pants themselves do not cause irritation; nevertheless, they retain both the heat given off by the body and the urine, which may produce irritation. Protective pants save time and money by cutting down on the amount of diaper changes necessary; however, the mother must be careful not to leave them on too long without changing the diaper.

Care of the baby in hot weather. In summer, babies require more fluids and should be offered plenty of water to drink. The need for solids diminishes and the baby may seem less hungry. Since fats produce heat, the baby's diet should contain less fat than during the winter.

In hot weather, if the baby vomits or has loose stools, all food must be stopped immediately and boiled skimmed milk substituted for the formula. If the symptoms cease, the formula may be given again in weakened amounts until full strength is attained. When older children have stomach upsets, fluids—juices, weak

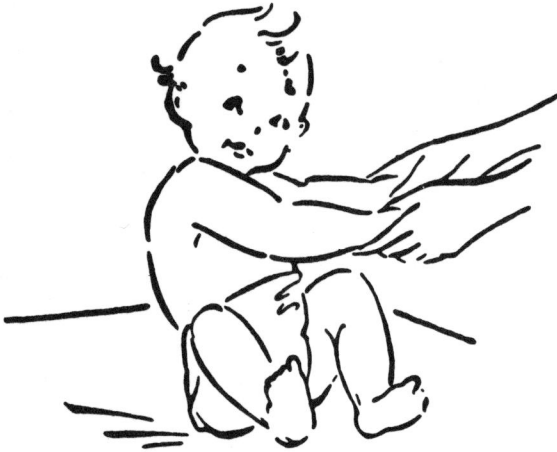

Baby Exercise 1 — The baby is laid on his back with his feet toward the mother. The mother then grasps the baby's hands and pulls him toward her. The exercise should be repeated two or three times. The baby tries to help himself up, which strengthens the arm, shoulder, neck, and abdominal muscles.

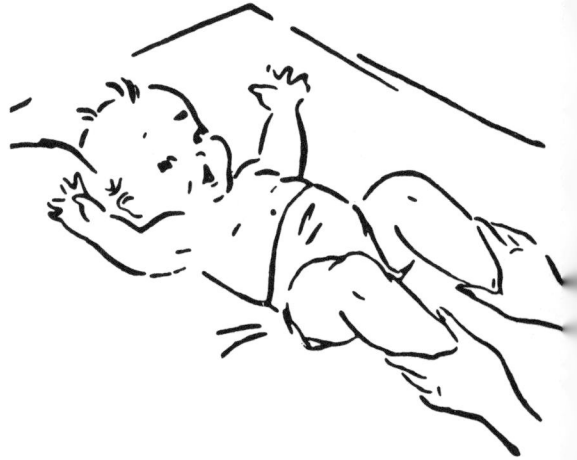

Exercise 2 — The baby is laid on his back with his feet toward the mother. The mother then grasps both feet and gently resists any movements that the baby may make. This resistance usually stimulates the baby to kick all the more. The exercise should be continued one or two minutes. It serves to strengthen the leg muscles.

tea, skimmed milk, clear soup—only are to be given.

During the summer, a baby can be clothed in very thin cotton underclothes and diapers. He will need more clothing early in the morning and late in the afternoon. A cotton sunsuit is sufficient clothing for a hot day. The baby's clothing should be a little lighter in hot weather than an adult's.

If the baby's skin is moist in hot weather, he is probably wearing too many clothes; and if his lips, fingers, and toes are cold, he needs more clothing.

Frequent baths are comforting to the baby in hot weather. The bath water should be tepid, not cold. One teaspoonful of baking soda to a pint of water soothes and helps cool the skin. After the bath, the baby may be powdered lightly. Cornstarch is as good as any other powder.

Exposure to sun. Moderate exposure to the sun is not dangerous to the baby's eyes or skin. In summer, the baby may take a nap in the sunlight in the morning or late in the afternoon, avoiding the extreme of heat at midday. Exposure to sun should be gradual, beginning with

Ulcers Of The Digestive Tract

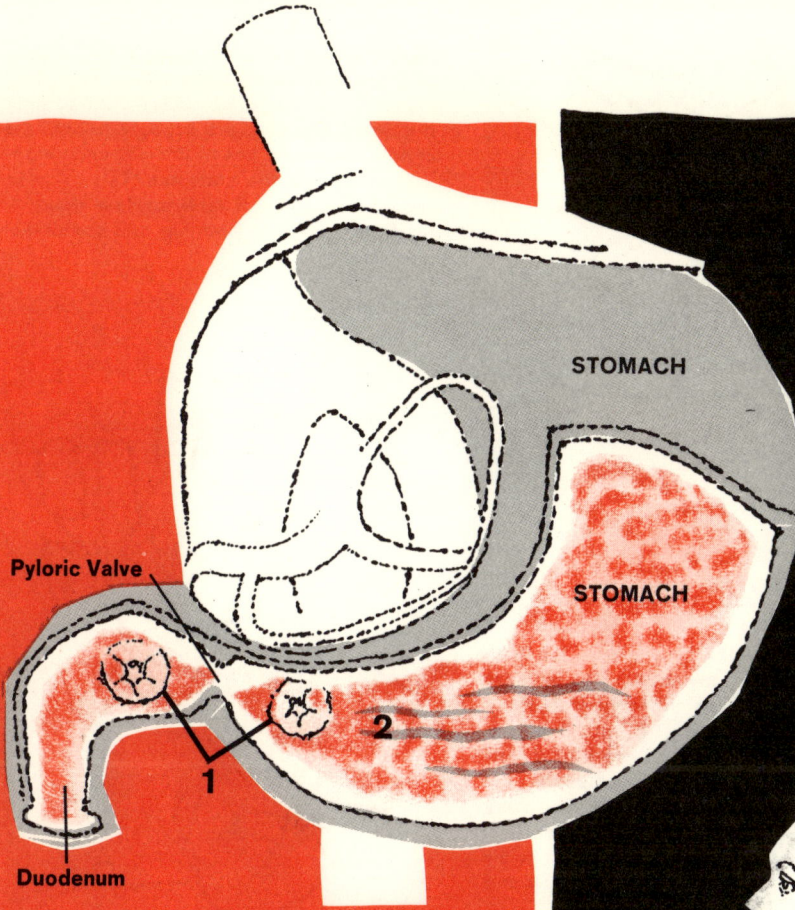

STOMACH

STOMACH

Pyloric Valve

2

1

Duodenum

3. Pain from stomach and duodenal ulcers frequently occurs in area outlined, and may go through to back. Has burning or gnawing character. But many ulcer patients experience pain in other areas of abdomen — or feel no apparent pain, though ulcer has developed.

1. Ulcers of digestive tract occur most often in stomach and upper part of small intestine (duodenum). Ulcer is open sore on inner surface of these organs. Without treatment, ulcer may hemorrhage, or eat through stomach or intestinal wall (perforated ulcer).

2. Higher than normal production of acid by stomach, while producing digestive juices, is one important cause of ulcers. Acid eats into lining of stomach and duodenum.

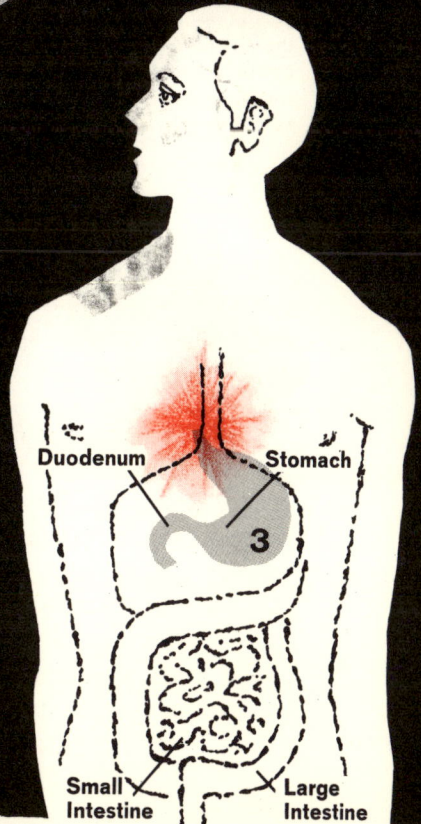

Duodenum   **Stomach**

3

Small Intestine   **Large Intestine**

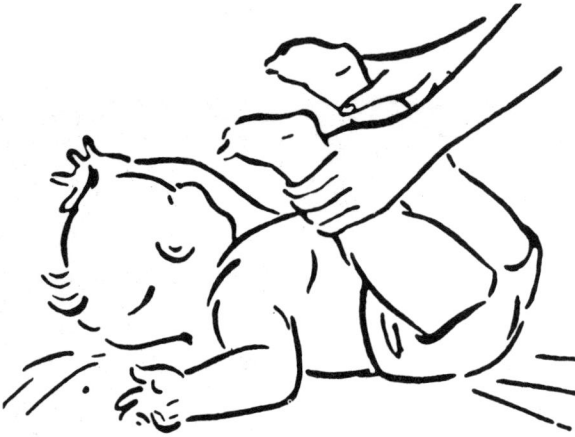

Exercise 3 — The baby is laid on his back with his feet toward the mother. The baby's legs are raised and the calves grasped near the ankle. The feet are brought toward the child's nose with knees straight and thighs in contact with the abdomen. This exercise should be repeated three or four times. It tends to strengthen both leg and abdominal muscles.

Exercise 4 — The baby is laid on his back with his feet toward the mother. The legs are grasped by the mother midway between the knees and the ankles. The legs then are raised until body and legs are almost vertical, with only the baby's head and upper part of the shoulders on the table. The baby then is returned to his original position. The exercise should be repeated two or three times. It tends to strengthen the trunk and spinal muscles.

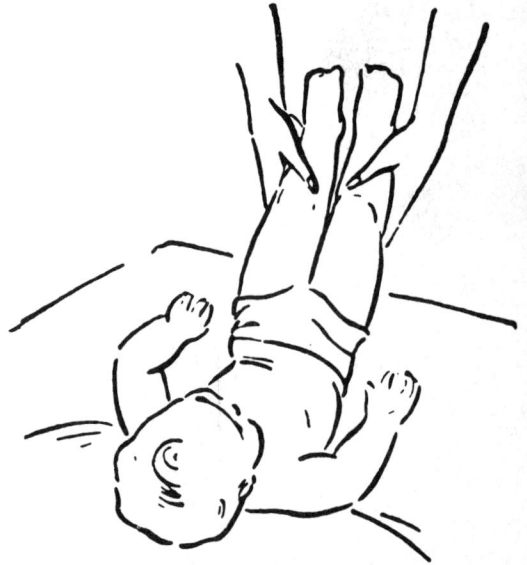

just a few minutes and increasing to about half an hour in direct exposure. A child may become ill or sunburned if exposure to sun is excessive. Various lotions are available which help to prevent an excessive reaction to the sun.

Traveling with the baby. Travel is not recommended or desirable for a very young baby. But short trips are often possible when the baby is slightly older and, if adequately planned in advance, can be done with a minimum of difficulty.

Car beds are obtainable and can be placed in the back seat of an automobile or taken on a train, bus, plane, or ship. They provide a comfortable resting or sleeping place for the baby. Extra diapers, fresh water, and canned formula or evaporated milk should be taken along in case of emergency. Refrigeration for the baby's formula bottles is sometimes possible on trains and other public transportation. If refrigeration is not available, a thermos bottle is a handy container for juice, formula, and other drinks for the baby, or an ice container may be used to keep the drinks cold.

Travel will be less taxing for the

Cancer of the Colon and Rectum

Right Side Cancer

Left Side Cancer

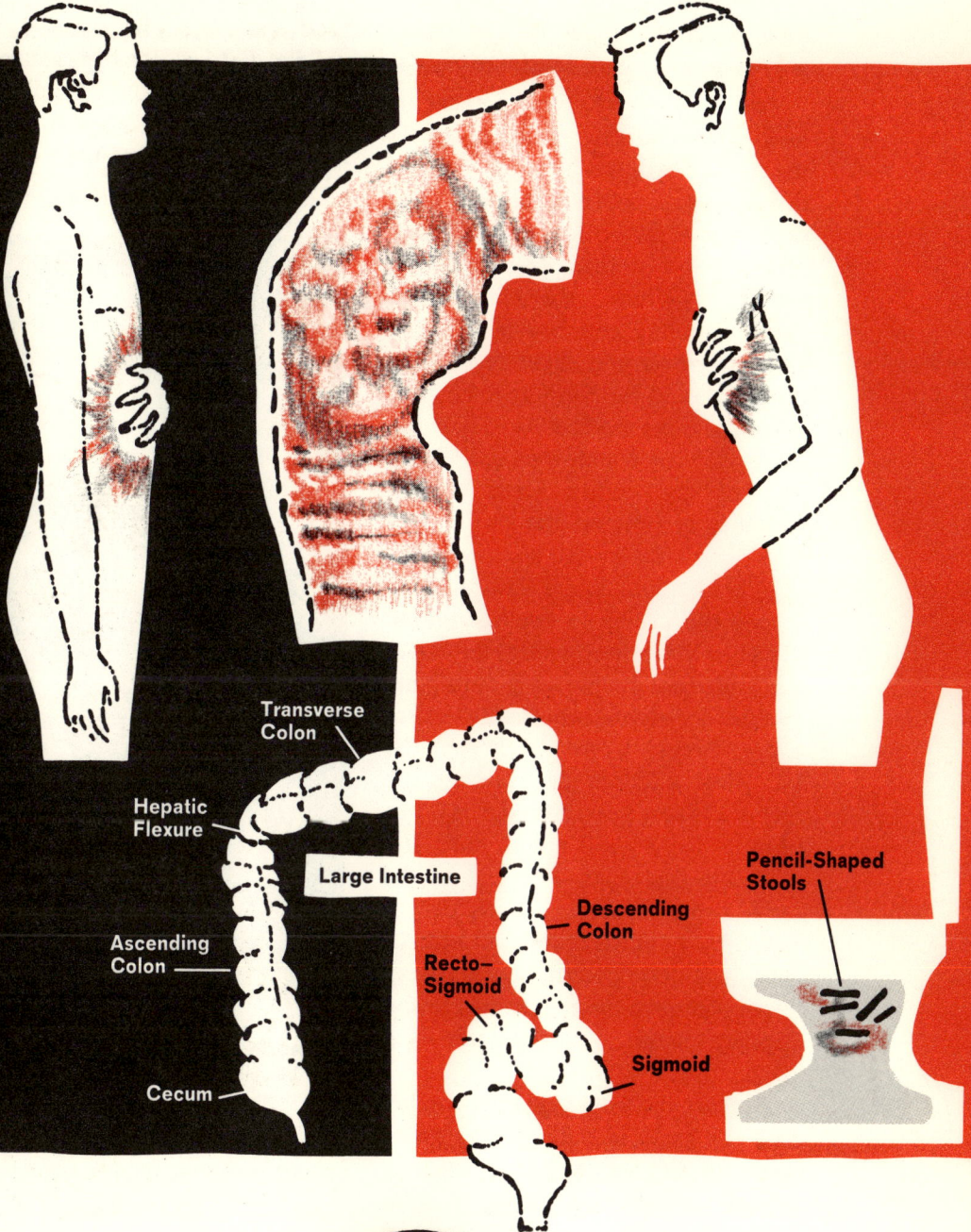

Transverse Colon

Hepatic Flexure

Large Intestine

Ascending Colon

Cecum

Descending Colon

Recto–Sigmoid

Sigmoid

Pencil-Shaped Stools

1. Weakness, fatigue, pain like appendicitis, anemia.

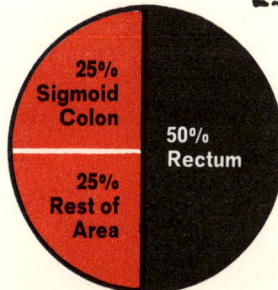

25% Sigmoid Colon

50% Rectum

25% Rest of Area

Obstruction of the bowel, leading to:

1. Alternating diarrhea and constipation, plus gassiness and abdominal pain

2. Blood mixed with mucus appears in stool. Stool changes to pencil shape

mother and child if it is done at a time when the roads or the transportation system is least congested.

The child's teeth. Development of teeth differs among children, as do the time of eruption and the reaction to teething. Even very healthy children may become fretful, sleep poorly, and refuse meals during teething periods. Teething often causes drooling of saliva, and looseness of bowels and slight fever. The doctor should be consulted; he may prescribe some medication to ease the baby over the teething period. Eruption of the child's teeth usually proceeds as follows: the two central lower teeth during the sixth to ninth month; the four upper central teeth during the eighth to twelfth month; the other two lower central teeth and the four front double teeth during the twelfth to eighteenth month. Altogether twenty teeth are in the first set. Most children have six by the end of the first year, although it is not unusual for a child not to have any teeth the first year. The rest of the teeth come between the eighteenth and twenty-fourth month, except the four back double teeth, which usually appear between the twenty-fourth and thirtieth month, but may come even later.

Because the teeth begin to form before the child is born, the pregnant woman's diet should be nutritionally adequate, including sufficient vitamins, minerals, especially calcium which is found in milk, and fresh vegetables, eggs, cooked fruits, cereals. Calcium supplements are often recommended.

To build healthy teeth, adequate food materials are essential in the child's diet, especially calcium and phosphorus, and the vitamins A, C, and D. The diet should include a sufficient quantity of milk each day, or its equivalent in butter or cheese,

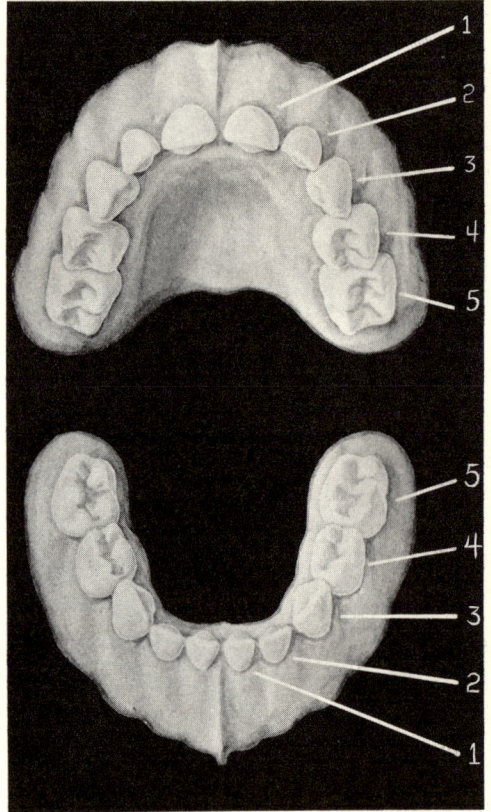

Child Care — The teeth must not be overlooked in child care. Many dental diseases can be prevented if the child is brought to the dentist regularly even though dental attention seems unnecessary. The first set of teeth are called deciduous, commonly known as milk teeth or baby teeth. These teeth are twenty in number and are smaller than the second set of teeth. Photograph shows the upper and lower jaws of a set of deciduous teeth. Upper jaw: (1) central incisor, (2) lateral incisor, (3) cuspid, (4) first molar, and (5) second molar. Lower jaw: (5) second molar, (4) first molar, (3) cuspid, (2) lateral incisor, and (1) central incisor.

Cancer of the Stomach

1. May develop anywhere in stomach. But cancers blocking entrance from esophagus **(A)** or exit to small intestine **(B)** give more clear cut early signs, are easier to diagnose.

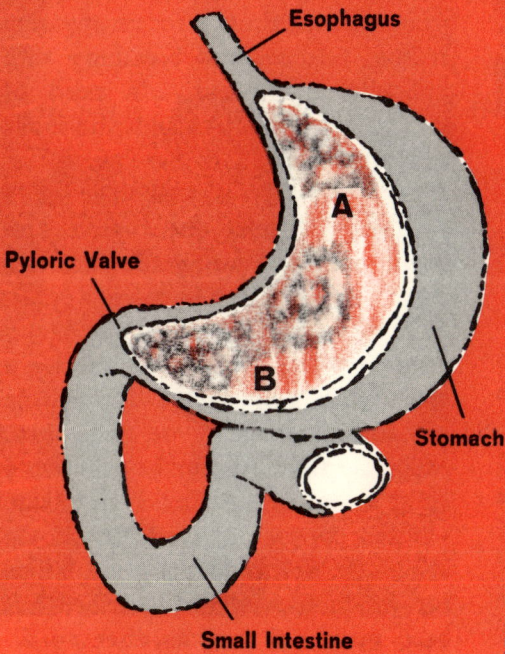

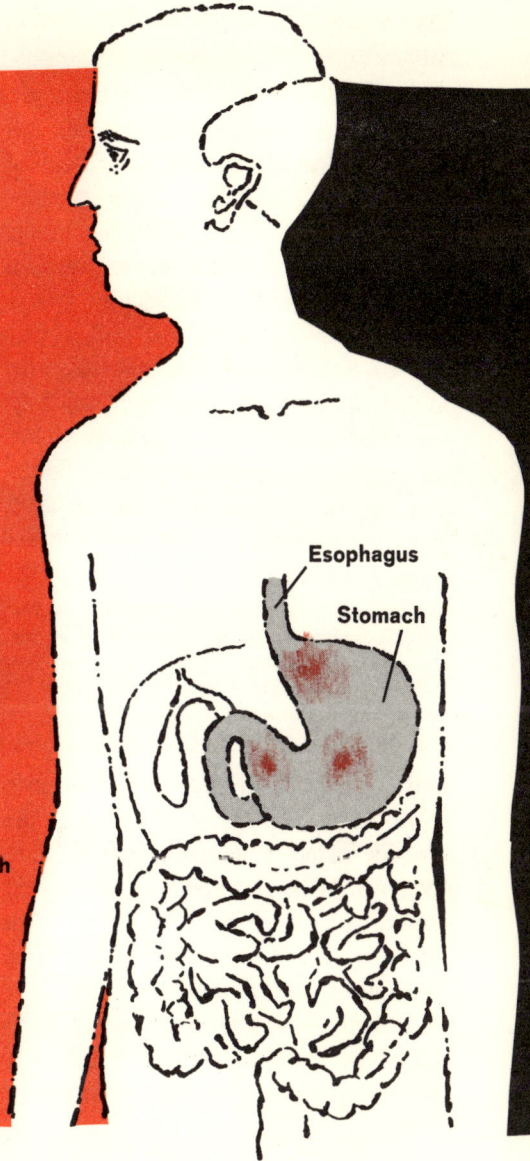

Esophagus

A

Pyloric Valve

B

Stomach

Small Intestine

Esophagus

Stomach

2. General symptoms: loss of weight, strength, appetite (particularly for meat), fullness and gas after eating, discomfort over abdomen. In later stages fully developed cancer can be felt through abdominal wall.

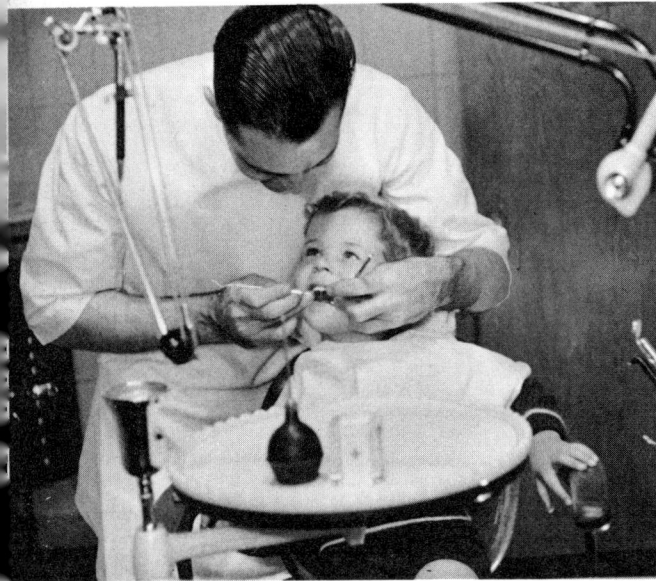

Child Care — Regular trips to visit the dentist are a pleasure for this child. He enjoys the kind attention and is interested in all the instruments and equipment. A healthy attitude toward good care of his teeth is being developed early.

and eggs, leafy green vegetables, and fresh fruit. For growing babies, the diet is often supplemented by cod liver oil. Milk and cheese are the best source of calcium. Foods rich in vitamin A are eggs, butter, carrots, and other vegetables. Vitamin C is abundant in citrus fruits, and D is found in fortified milk, in cod liver oil, and in most vitamin preparations.

Many physicians feel that coarse foods strengthen the jaws and help to harden the gums. When a new tooth is coming in, coarse foods serve as a resistance against which the gums may work to permit the teeth to cut their way through. Heredity is also significant in determining the type and quality of the child's teeth.

Special mouth care is not essential during the first two years. Some time in the beginning of the third year the child may be shown how to use a toothbrush by having him imitate the actions of the older person. During his third year the child should see a dentist, who will note any difficulties and plan for future care.

The sick child. Since children are not as articulate in drawing attention to their needs as adults, most mothers soon learn how to detect the first signs of illness. The child who is listless, drowsy for no apparent reason, flushed, and breathing with difficulty is obviously in need of medical attention. A child who looks and acts well and has plenty of energy probably is well. The child should get regular checkups at frequent intervals during the first two years, and after that twice a year. Most communities have public health services where a child may receive a checkup without charge if a private pediatrician cannot be consulted. Medicine should never be given to a child unless ordered by a physician. Unused portions of medicine should always be destroyed after the illness for which they were prescribed has been cured. If, months after an illness, the child develops what seems to be the "same" condition, under no circumstances should he be given the original prescription unless ordered by a doctor.

The child in the hospital. If a child must be hospitalized, for an operation or a protracted stay, there are a number of things to know and to be done which can help the child through the experience. The child

Ulcerative Colitis

1. Fever

2. Loss of appetite and weight

3. Diarrhea

4. Bright red blood and mucus in bowel movement

5. Inflammation and ulcers visible on doctor's proctoscopic and x-ray examination

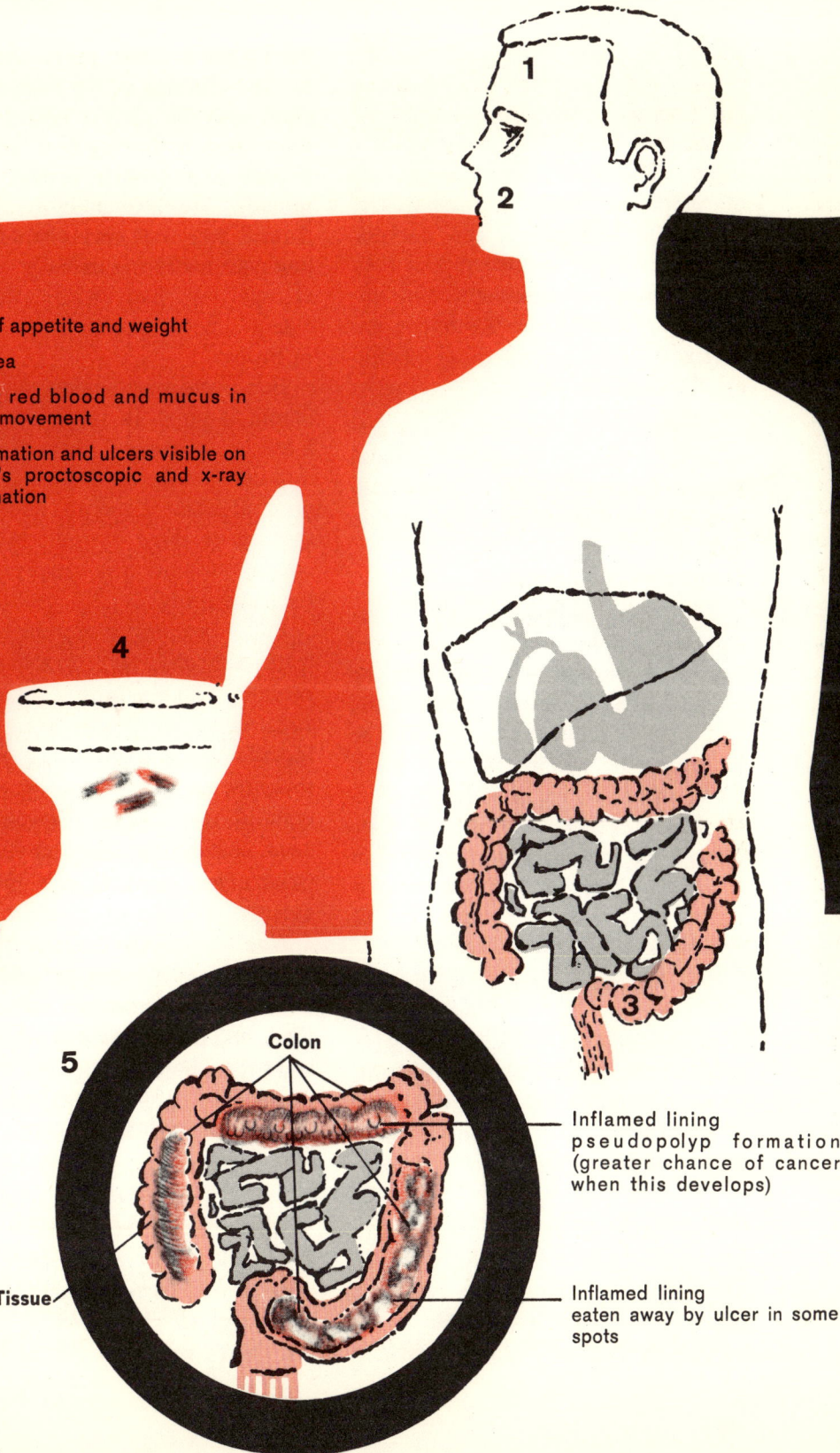

Colon

Normal Tissue

Inflamed lining pseudopolyp formation (greater chance of cancer when this develops)

Inflamed lining eaten away by ulcer in some spots

should be intelligently prepared for his stay in the hospital. Confidence in the doctors and nurses should be established by suitable explanations; visits to the child planned as periods of happiness rather than of worry. The child will reflect his parents' attitudes so it is important that they appear hopeful, confident, and encouraging throughout the entire experience. The homecoming should also be carefully planned.

Prevention of infection. Some diseases can be prevented by inoculation or vaccination, including smallpox, diphtheria, whooping cough, scarlet fever, measles, typhoid fever, tetanus, and poliomyelitis.

Although smallpox is rare nowadays, every child should be vaccinated against it, and in most parts of the country this is mandatory before the child can be admitted to school. The child may be vaccinated when he is from three to six months of age. Ordinarily vaccination is not done during the summer months, and it should be postponed if the child is not well or if other children in the family have infectious diseases.

Vaccination is best performed on the outer side of the upper arm. Although many parents of baby girls demand vaccination on the thigh, this is not always a safe technique because of difficulty in keeping the area clean and free of infection.

Usually, after a week, a small pimple forms at the site of the vaccination and in a few days the area around the vaccination may swell and become black and blue. This is the normal process of a vaccination and

should not cause alarm. The vaccination must be kept dry until the crust falls off. To prevent scratching the area, the child may wear a long-sleeved shirt day and night. Occasionally the vaccination will not "take," and must be repeated. Smallpox vaccination is usually repeated at age six, just before the child enters school, and again at the age of twelve.

For protection against diphtheria, toxoid is given in three doses, once a month, starting at the age of three months. Booster injections should be given at eighteen months and again at the age of three or four. Whooping cough vaccination is usually given at the same time.

Polio vaccination should be given when the child is six months old, repeated two weeks to a month later and again in about six months. Inoculations against other illnesses, such as measles, scarlet fever, and typhoid fever, can be given as the need arises according to the physician's judgment of the individual case.

Hygiene for the sick child. If the child has an infectious disease, all unnecessary draperies, carpets, pictures, and other articles such as books and toys should be removed from the sickroom before the child is put into it. Occasionally, in a serious illness, objects with which the child has been in contact must be destroyed. Hardwood or metal pieces of furniture are preferable for the sickroom rather than stuffed furniture, because they are easier to clean. When possible, the child's room should be near the

Cirrhosis of the Liver

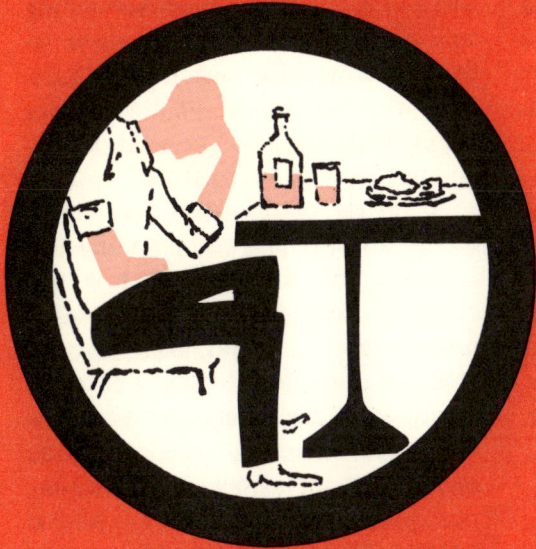

◀ **Early Stage**

Weak, tired feeling

Nausea, vomiting

Constipation or diarrhea

Loss of appetite

Frequently consequence of alcoholism

Advanced Stage ▶

Jaundice (yellowing of skin and eye balls)

Broken blood vessels

Enlargement of male breasts

Hardened, lumpy liver

Swelling of abdomen

Enlarged veins around navel

Loss of pubic and armpit hair

Shrinking of testicles—impotence

Patchy inflammation of palms

Large blood spots

Swelling of ankles

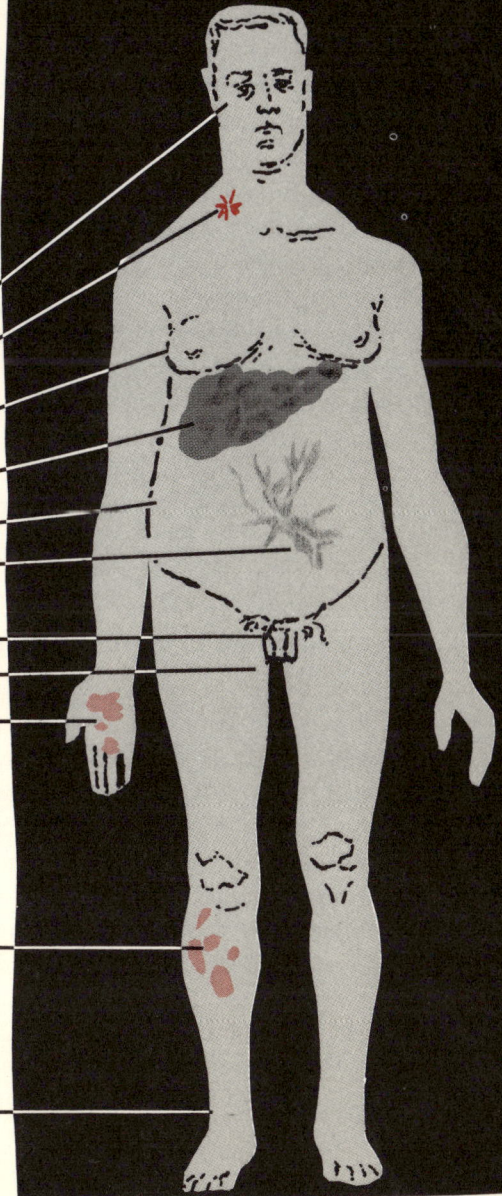

bathroom to lessen the amount of work.

The person who cares for a child with an infectious disease should wear a washable smock over her clothing. She should also wear a cloth mask and wash her hands thoroughly after leaving the child.

A large paper bag is useful at the side of the sick child's bed. In this can be placed soiled towels, used gauze, cotton, and other sickroom items. The entire bag and its contents can then be conveniently disposed of daily. If the infection is contagious, it is best to burn the waste.

The sick child should be dressed in a loose-fitting, easily washable garment and the room should be well ventilated, although free from unusually cold drafts. Bathing the sick child is preferably done by a careful sponge bath rather than immersion in a tub. After the sponge bath, the child may receive an alcohol rub, or, if he is too young for this, talcum or cornstarch may be patted over his body. If the child has much fever, cold cream or petroleum jelly applied to the lips helps to overcome dryness and crusting.

Fever. A fever usually indicates that the child is ill, although occasionally a slight variation in temperature is not a sign of illness. Every parent should know how to read a thermometer and both rectal and oral thermometers should be on hand in the medicine chest. A small child's temperature is best taken with a rectal thermometer. The normal range is between 99° and 100° when taken rectally (usually one degree

higher than an oral temperature). To be certain of a correct reading, the thermometer must be shaken down well and left in position for three to five minutes. After use, it should be washed in lukewarm, not hot, water, rinsed with alcohol if possible, dried, and put away in a safe place.

A variety of disorders may cause elevations of temperature in children. Simplest and most common is the ordinary cold, which may give a high temperature. A sore throat, stomach upset, or infection will cause fever, as will the onset of the common childhood diseases, scarlet fever, measles, whooping cough, or chickenpox. When the temperature is above normal, the doctor should be consulted and no home treatment, such as laxatives or enemas, should be given until they are prescribed.

Many feverish babies feel better after a sponge bath with lukewarm water. Ice-cold rub-downs or alcohol should not be given to babies under two years of age. Occasionally the doctor may order a cool-water enema for a high temperature, or prescribe a small dose of aspirin. These treatments are soothing, but usually do not cure the cause of the rise in temperature. The doctor should always be consulted about what to feed the sick child. In most instances a poor appetite follows a high temperature and parents should not force the child to eat. Fluids may be encouraged, but solids are to be avoided during the first few days of the illness.

The common cold. The most frequent illness in babies is the common cold. It is usually not serious, even

Amebiasis and Amebic Dysentery

Caused by Amebae (microscopic-sized one cell animals)

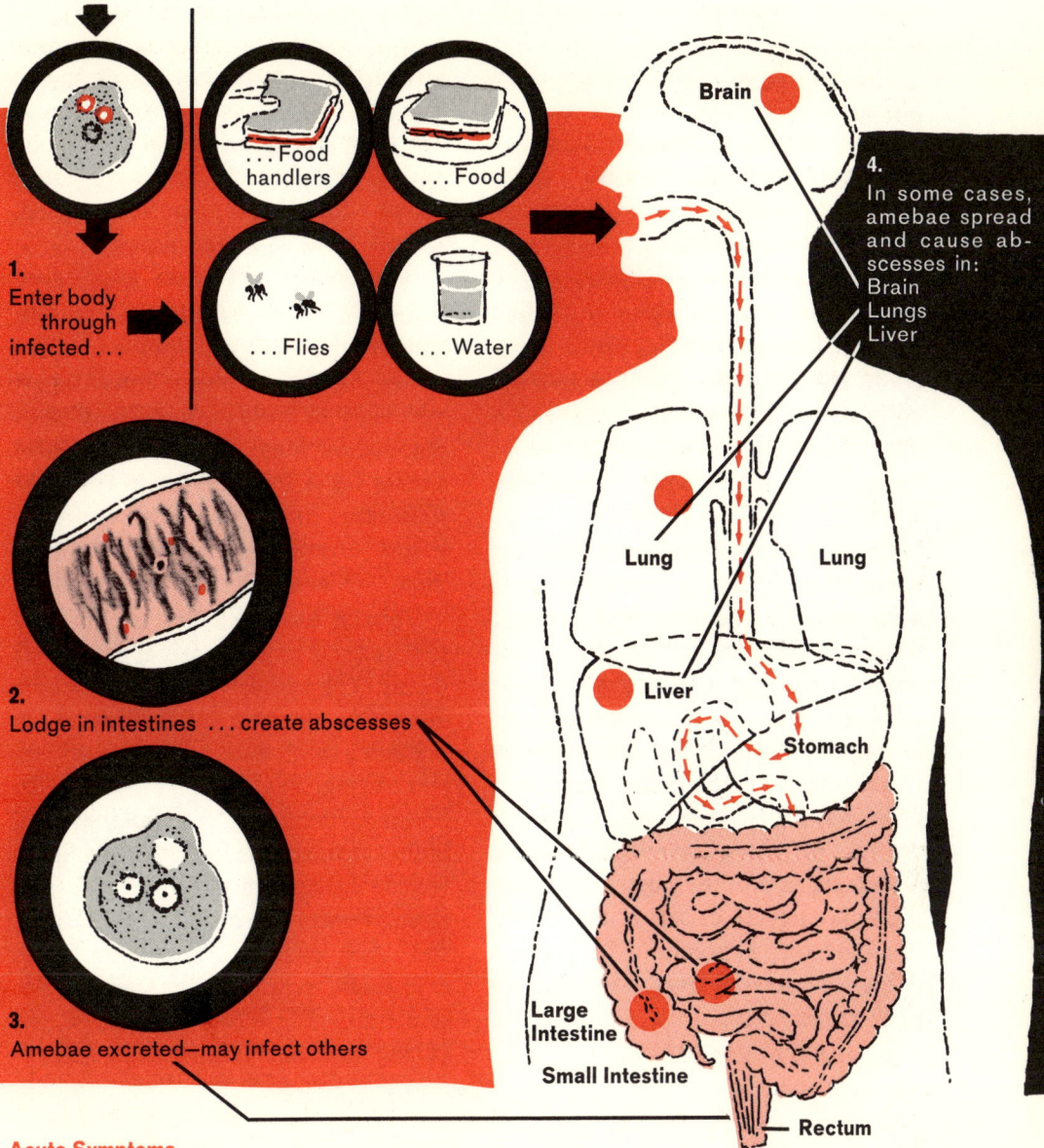

1. Enter body through infected . . .

. . . Food handlers

. . . Food

. . . Flies

. . . Water

2. Lodge in intestines . . . create abscesses

3. Amebae excreted—may infect others

Brain

4. In some cases, amebae spread and cause abscesses in: Brain Lungs Liver

Lung

Lung

Liver

Stomach

Large Intestine

Small Intestine

Rectum

Acute Symptoms

Abdominal pains, nausea, vomiting

Up to 15-20 liquid stools a day. Often contain blood and mucus

Doctor's miscroscopic examination of stool reveals amebae

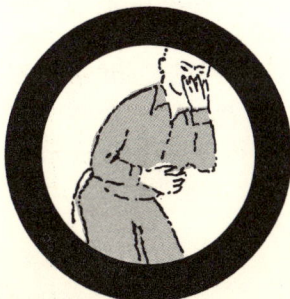

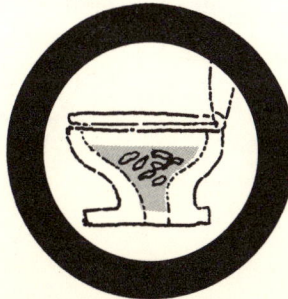

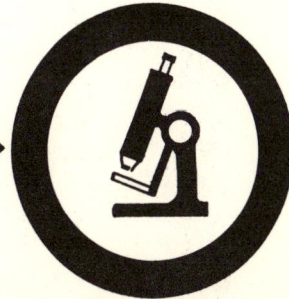

when the temperature is elevated, but because of the danger of the cold's developing complications such as pneumonia, bronchitis, or ear infection, the doctor should be called promptly. The best way to avoid contracting colds is to avoid exposure to persons with colds. Other factors, such as chilling, poor nutrition, and fatigue are probably also significant in making the child more prone to the cold. The child with a cold is more comfortable in a moist environment. This does not mean a damp room, but rather a properly humidified room.

Enlarged tonsils and adenoids seem to make children more susceptible to sore throat. If the tonsils are found to be infected, the doctor should decide whether or not they should be removed.

Babies may have tub baths in winter, but the room in which it is given should be warm and free from drafts. A brisk, gentle rub-down afterward is also helpful. Preferably the bath is given at night, just before the baby goes to bed.

Use of vaccines to prevent colds is as yet not established as effective. Nose drops may be prescribed to clear the nasal passages and permit easier respiration. At the first sign of a cold with nasal drip, cough, or rise of temperature, the child should be put to bed, and his food intake lessened. If the child runs a fever, of more than 102°, the doctor should be called.

Hernia. Frequently a child is born with a weak spot in the muscles of the belly wall or groin. This condition is commonly known as a rupture or hernia. Swelling is caused when the intestines or other tissues are pushed through the weak spot in the wall. Often the spot appears around the navel in newborn babies. When the child coughs, cries, or strains, the rupture is seen more easily because of the increased pressure within the abdominal cavity. Usually the lump disappears on lying down. Operation is not immediately necessary in these instances and often the doctor may just tape the navel hernia for a few months in the hope that scar tissue will seal over the defect. Hernias in the groin are less likely to disappear without surgery.

Tonsils and adenoids. Apparently tonsils serve to take care of infectious germs. The tonsils frequently become inflamed, swollen, and infected in children, and may cause pain on swallowing, earache, difficulty in hearing, breathing, or talking, and high temperature. The organism which causes most tonsillitis, the streptococcus, is similar to the organism that leads to rheumatic fever, erysipelas, scarlet fever, and other disorders. Penicillin is effective in curing tonsillitis in most cases and removal is not always necessary unless sore throats are particularly recurrent or resistant to penicillin, or the tonsils are enlarged.

The child with tonsillitis should remain in bed. If he is able to gargle, salt water will help to shrink the throat tissues. An ice collar and aspirin may give relief of pain. The doctor may use injections of penicillin or pills to help cure the infection,

Appendicitis and Peritonitis

1. Appendicitis . . .

A. In typical cases, starts with off-and-on pain near navel.

B. Pain radiates down to right lower abdomen over appendix. Becomes constant and progressively more severe. Spot is tender to touch.

C. Nausea and occasionally vomiting follows. Sequence may take anywhere from several hours to 1-2 days.

D. Blood test reveals inflammation.

E. Attack may pass by itself. But if it gets worse . . .

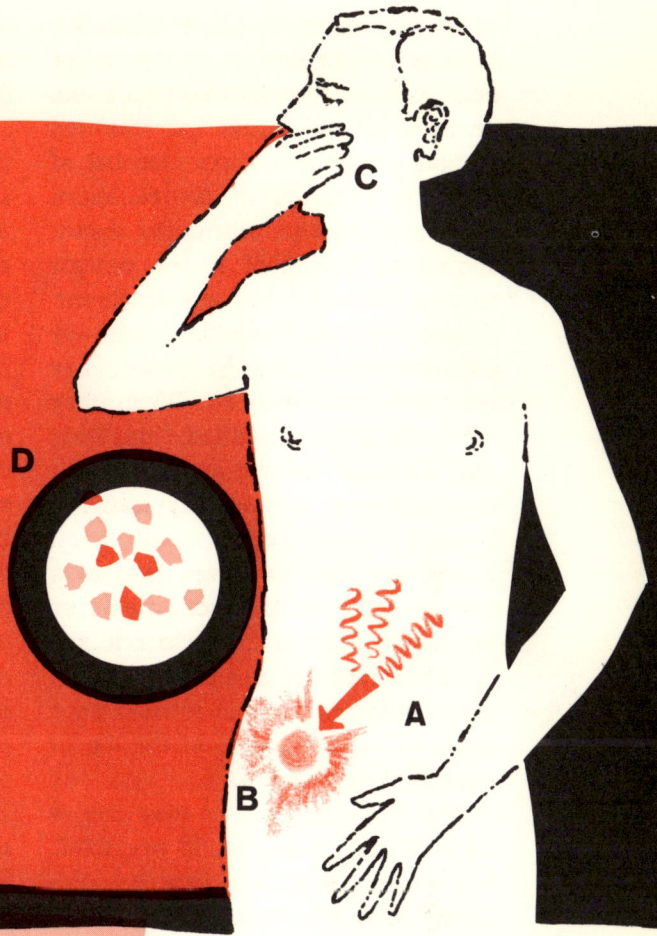

2. . . . and Peritonitis

. . . infection from badly inflamed or bursting appendix may spread to peritoneum (membrane lining of abdomen). Resulting peritonitis may severely infect whole abdominal area.

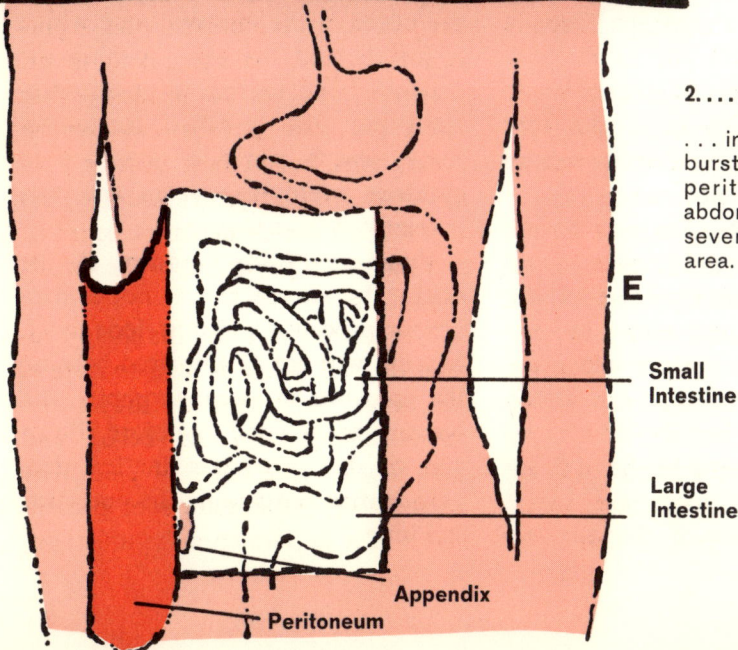

Small Intestine

Large Intestine

Appendix

Peritoneum

or he may prescribe other medicines such as Terramycin, Achromycin, or one of the other antibiotics. These drugs must never be administered without a doctor's orders. Because of the serious nature of complications from neglected tonsillitis, the doctor should be consulted if the parents suspect the child has a sore throat.

The adenoids lie in the cavity behind the nose. Like the tonsils, they are prone to infections. When they are enlarged or infected, breathing and talking is difficult and the child's voice has a nasal twang. Typically he keeps his mouth open at all times. Eventually this may even lead to a change in facial expression; the upper lip is shortened and turned out, the lips are thickened, and a line between the cheeks and lips is formed as a result of the narrowing of the dental arch of the upper jaw.

Infections of the ear may follow adenoid infection and, if neglected, can lead to permanent deafness. Enlarged adenoids should be removed; this may be done at any age. Usually further trouble will not be encountered after tonsils and adenoids are removed, but in 10 to 15 per cent of cases they grow back and a second operation may be required.

Care of the ears. The ears do not require special care. Syringes should not be used to wash out the ears, nor should cotton-tipped sticks be employed to remove wax or other objects. When a small child has a pain in his ear, he will usually indicate his discomfort by putting his hand to his ear or by crying when the ear is touched. Infections of the ear frequently follow infectious conditions in the nose or throat and acute infectious diseases.

When the doctor examines the child with a painful ear, he routinely takes the temperature, which is usually quite high, even in simple ear infections. Next he will look directly into the ear canal with a special instrument, the otoscope. If infection is present, and the condition warrants, the doctor may make a small opening in the eardrum to release accumulations of fluid or pus. Otherwise, simple antibiotic treatment may be all that is required. Relief of pain is usually prompt following drainage or other therapy. Sometimes the pain of earache may be relieved by ear drops prescribed by the physician. Such treatment should not be used unless a doctor has seen the child.

Before the introduction of penicillin, ear infections often caused more or less permanent deafness. Mastoid infection too was frequent. In mastoid infection, severe pain and tenderness are noted in the mastoid bone which is just behind the ear. Opening the mastoid bone to free it of accumulated pus, the so-called mastoidectomy, was a common operation in children twenty-five years ago, but is relatively rare today.

Puncture of the eardrum by the doctor to release pus is not a dangerous procedure. If it is done early, hearing will not be impaired because the eardrum will heal promptly and hearing be as good as before. Puncture of the eardrum is far less dangerous than postponing the operation too long.

410

Cancer of the Pancreas

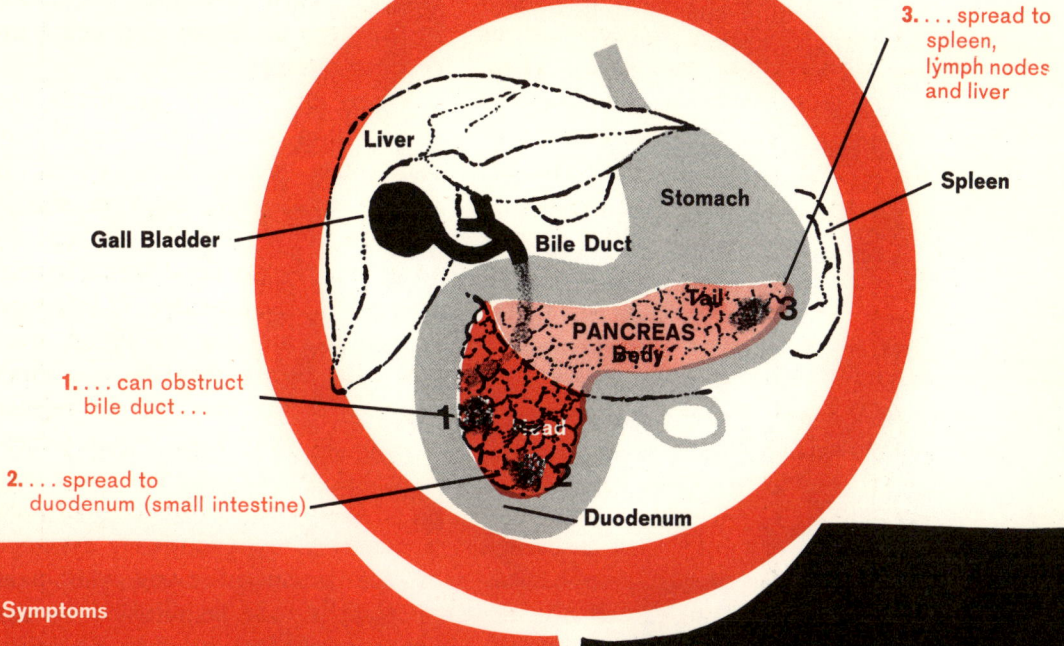

3. . . . spread to spleen, lymph nodes and liver

Liver

Gall Bladder

Stomach

Bile Duct

Spleen

Tail

PANCREAS
Body

1. . . . can obstruct bile duct . . .

Head

2. . . . spread to duodenum (small intestine)

Duodenum

Symptoms

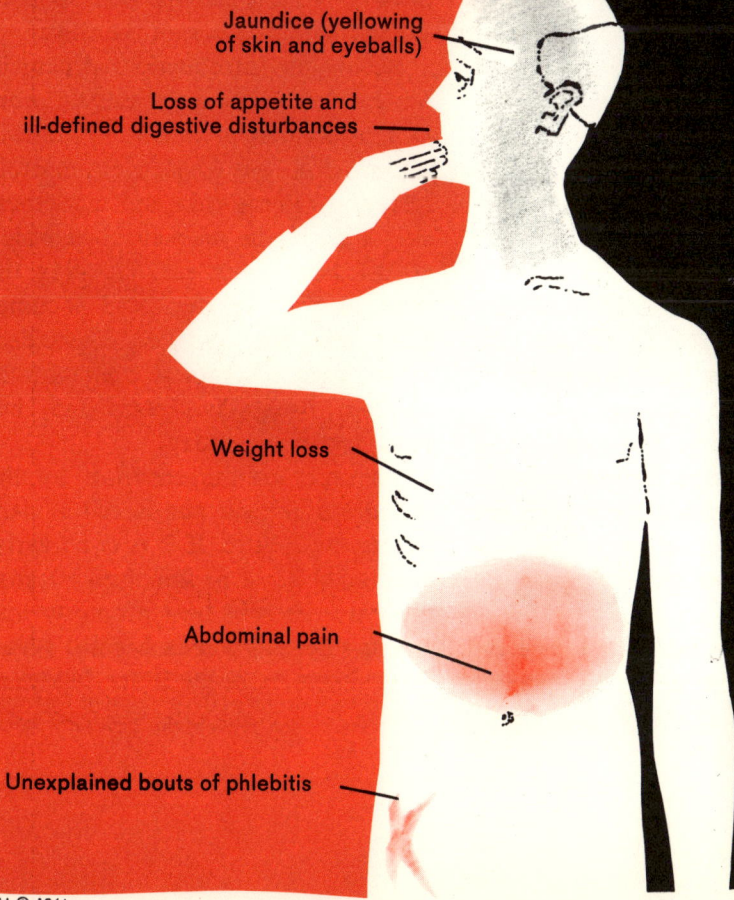

Jaundice (yellowing of skin and eyeballs)

Loss of appetite and ill-defined digestive disturbances

Weight loss

Abdominal pain

Unexplained bouts of phlebitis

Cuts and bruises. Little children frequently suffer cuts, bruises, burns, and similar injuries to the skin which can possibly become infected. In such instances, first aid given at home is of the greatest significance in preventing complications from simple injuries. Many different antiseptic substances are available to kill germs located on the skin around a skin injury. The area affected should be washed immediately with plenty of soap and water. A suitable antiseptic may then be applied, but a clean cut usually requires only a finger-bandage such as the Band-Aid. Children often object to iodine solutions or alcohol because of the burning sensation, and other non-burning antiseptics may be used.

Occasionally a bruise to the finger-tips may result in a painful swollen area of blood clot under the nail. The doctor should be called. Most likely he will make a small nick in the nail to permit free drainage and relief from pain. This should never be done by anyone but a physician. Bruises which are painful often can be relieved from pain by cold compresses.

Convulsions in babies. Babies have convulsions much more frequently than adults. The nervous system of

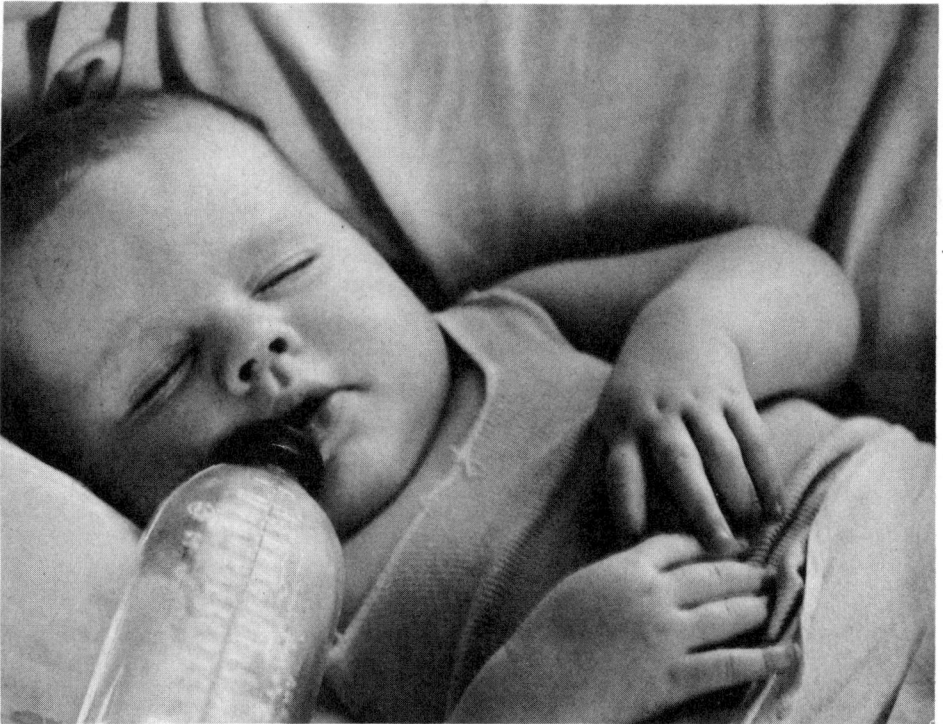

Child Care — Permitting the child to sleep with the nursing bottle in the mouth may deform the face. Later in life facial disfigurements are of great psychological importance. Bad eating and sleeping habits which may cause deformity of the face or malocclusion should be interrupted as soon as possible. Good care and close supervision can prevent the development of these habits.

a baby is so sensitive that frequently an infectious disease or high temperature will give rise to a convulsion or extensive shaking. In ordinary convulsions, the child loses consciousness and becomes rigid. Then there may be a spasmodic jerking of the face and of the arms and legs. It may be difficult for the parent to differentiate between a simple convulsion and one due to epilepsy. In only about one-fifth of convulsions in children is the cause epilepsy. Convulsions should be promptly reported to the doctor. During a convulsion, the child should be placed gently on his side. Usually the child will sleep following a convulsion.

See also BED WETTING; COLIC; EYE; FEEDING, BREAST; HEAD BANGING, HEAD ROLLING; IMMUNIZATION; THUMB SUCKING.

CHILD CARE – adolescence: See article SEX HYGIENE, page 1681-89.

CHILD CARE – adoption: See article SEX HYGIENE, page 1698.

CHILD CARE – allergy: See article ALLERGY, pages 90-92, 94.

CHILD CARE – born after forty: See article SEX HYGIENE, page 1698.

CHILD CARE – cancer: See article CANCER, page 349-50.

CHILD CARE – chicken pox: See article INFECTIOUS DISEASES OF CHILDHOOD, page 1116-18.

CHILD CARE – curiosity regarding sex: See article SEX HYGIENE, page 1679-80.

CHILD CARE – diphtheria: See article INFECTIOUS DISEASES OF CHILDHOOD, page 1100-06.

CHILD CARE – diseases, infectious: See article INFECTIOUS DISEASES OF CHILDHOOD, page 1100-24.

CHILD CARE – eczema: See article ALLERGY, page 83-85.

CHILD CARE – exercise: See article SEX HYGIENE, page 1679-81.

CHILD CARE – German measles: See article INFECTIOUS DISEASES OF CHILDHOOD, page 1109-12.

CHILD CARE – half educated before starting to school: See article SEX HYGIENE, page 1681-82.

CHILD CARE – immunization procedures: See article ALLERGY, pages 92, 94.

CHILD CARE – infantile paralysis: See article INFECTIOUS DISEASES OF CHILDHOOD, page 1119-24.

CHILD CARE – infectious diseases: See article INFECTIOUS DISEASES OF CHILDHOOD, page 1100-24.

CHILD CARE – intussusception: See article DIGESTION AND DIGESTIVE DISEASES, page 901.

CHILD CARE – jealousy of newborn baby: See article CARE OF MOTHERS BEFORE AND AFTER CHILDBIRTH, page 1541.

CHILD CARE – love affairs: See article SEX HYGIENE, page 1678-80.

CHILD CARE – measles: See article INFECTIOUS DISEASES OF CHILDHOOD, page 1105-10.

CHILD CARE – mental training: See article NERVOUS AND MENTAL DISORDERS, page 1272.

CHILD CARE – mumps: See article INFECTIOUS DISEASES OF CHILDHOOD, page 1117-20.

CHILD CARE – posture exercises: See article POSTURE, page 1484.

CHILD CARE – pyelitis: See article THE KIDNEY: ITS DISEASES AND DISTURBANCES, page 1194.

CHILD CARE – rheumatic fever: See article DISEASES OF THE HEART AND CIRCULATION, pages 987-88, 990.

CHILD CARE – scarlet fever: See article INFECTIOUS DISEASES OF CHILDHOOD, page 1111-14.

CHILD CARE – self-control: See article SEX HYGIENE, page 1680-81.

CHILD CARE – skin care: See article THE SKIN, page 1745.

CHILD CARE – tuberculars should be sent away: See article THE RESPIRATORY DISEASES, page 1606.

CHILD CARE – whooping cough: See article INFECTIOUS DISEASES OF CHILDHOOD, page 1114-17.

CHILD CARE – young married couple and: See article SEX HYGIENE, page 1697-98.

what your baby needs from you in his
FIRST TWO YEARS

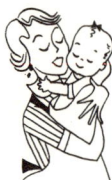

He needs to be carried often to develop his sense of balance and his feeling of security.

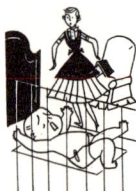

Giving the baby prompt attention when he cries develops his sense of safety and trust.

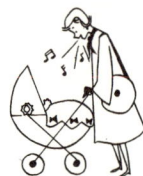

Singing, rocking, patting or holding your baby when he's wakeful helps him sleep.

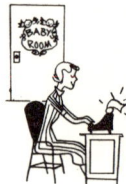

A room of his own is important for baby's quiet and comfort and your own privacy.

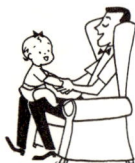

Companionship and play with parents are important to any baby.

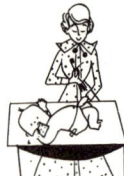

Needs matter-of-fact parental attitudes. Show no disgust at elimination.

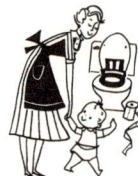

With a little help a child toilet trains himself when he is ready.

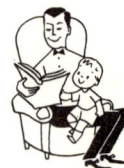

Needs practice in talking and listening, to develop his ability to communicate.

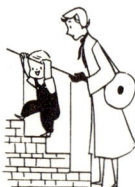

Needs to be given as much freedom as is sensible, not hedged in with Don'ts.

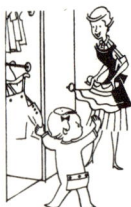

By asserting himself, he gains the sense of being an individual.

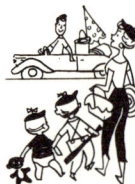

He also needs to feel that he is a member of a family group.

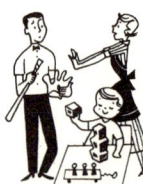

Among his needs are toys and materials he can master—not ones he can't manage.

Here's the first in a unique series of pictographs which depict the all-important needs of children as they grow from birth into the teens. These features are based on scientific studies and research

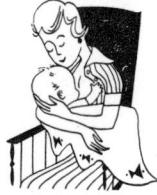

Baby needs mothering—being held and caressed—especially at feeding time.

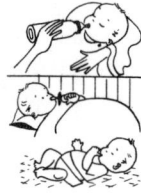

New baby needs several hours of sucking a day.

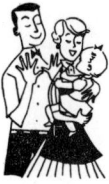

Needs frequent, open display of affection—since he learns to love by being loved.

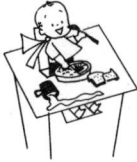

Let him feed himself when he shows interest—even though he makes a mess.

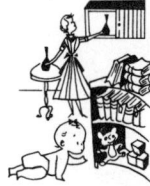

Be sure your baby has room and opportunity for free movement and exploration.

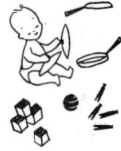

His first playthings should be ones that satisfy his need to handle, bang, suck, throw.

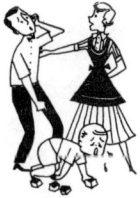

Needs to have his parents realize that he is not a little adult.

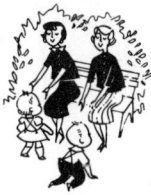

A child needs to grow at his own pace and be appreciated—not pushed.

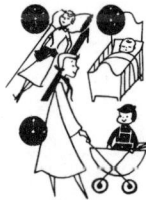

Needs a relaxed, responsive mother who plans rest and recreation for herself and her baby.

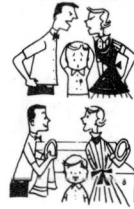

A cooperative, harmonious home atmosphere is important—tensions distress a baby.

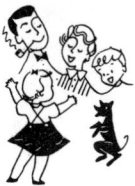

A child needs to be able and encouraged to display love for others.

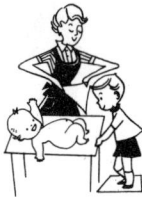

He needs to consider all parts of his body as clean and acceptable.

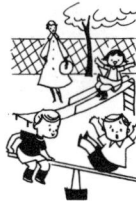

The young child needs to climb, run, pull, be physically active.

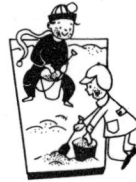

He needs to play freely and be allowed to get dirty.

Graphics Institute, N. Y. C.

Three is a delightful age. A child has greater self-control, is friendly and cooperative and learning to manage social relationships. Let's follow him through a typical day.

introducing the
THREE-YEAR-OLD

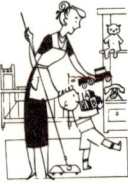

Will cooperate in clearing the table, tidying his own room— if asked.

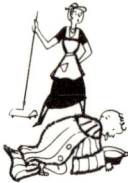

Sometimes creates imaginary playmates, pets, or pretends that he is an animal.

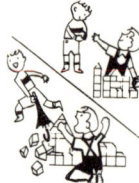

Alternates between pestering brothers and sisters, and getting along with them.

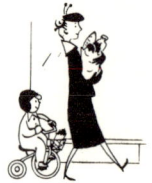

Learning to ride tricycle. Likes to go marketing with mother.

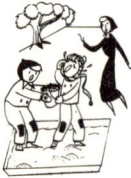

Needs guidance when play gets quarrelsome. Aggressiveness expressed in words as well as actions.

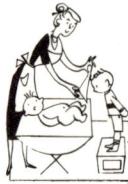

Notices sex differences and sometimes worries about them. Questions should be answered simply.

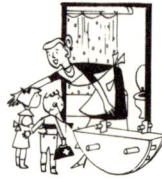

May handle genitals. Can be quite matter-of-factly distracted from sex play.

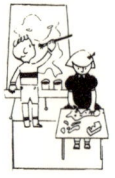

Likes to have familiar stories read without change. Enjoys explaining pictures.

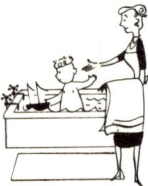

Likes to help prepare his bath, wash himself. Gets out unwillingly.

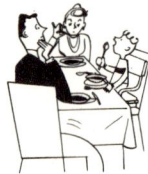

May try to be the center of attention if eating with family. Eats well by himself.

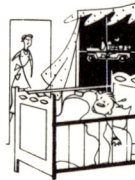

Outcropping fears: of the dark, dogs, other animals, fire engines. Needs reassurance.

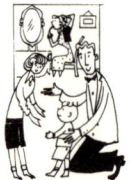

When he knows parents are going out may say good-bye cheerfully. Or may protest until older.

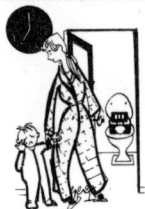

Frequently whines upon awakening. May drowse off after getting mother's help in toileting.

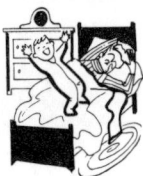

Cheers up when fully awake. Likes to frisk around parents' room and get dressed with them.

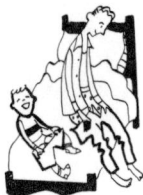

Can put on pants, socks, shoes, sweater. Able to undress easily, undo buttons —but can't button them.

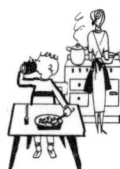

Appetite usually good for breakfast. Feeds himself skillfully—not much parental help is needed.

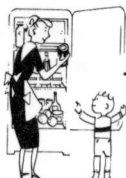

Requests favorite foods (such as fruit, meat, milk) when meal is being prepared.

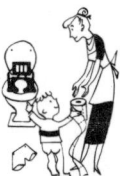

Gaining good control of elimination. Frequently has bowel movement after lunch.

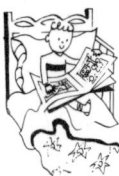

Willing to rest at naptime, but frequently does not go to sleep.

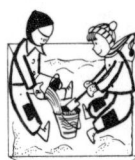

Beginning to be able to play with other children, as well as beside them. Has definite choice in friends.

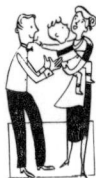

Affectionate toward parents. Mother is generally the favorite.

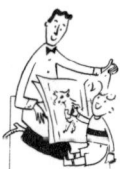

Enjoys painting, crayoning, modeling with clay. Results seldom resemble what he calls them.

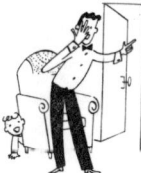

Welcomes playtime with his father. Likes riddles and enjoys guessing games.

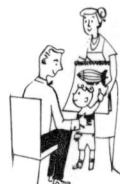

Listens to adults. Wants to please and enjoys praise. Likes to master new words.

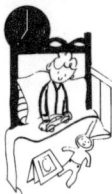

Plays in bed for half hour or so. Usually goes to sleep without too many demands.

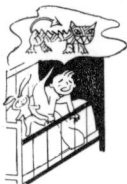

Begins to talk about his dreams and may occasionally be wakened in fright by nightmare.

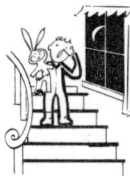

Frequently gets up during night. May get out of bed and wander around the house.

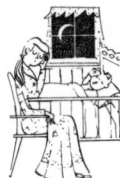

May want to get in bed with mother. But can usually be diverted if parent stays with him awhile.

a pictorial guide to the
FOUR-YEAR-OLD

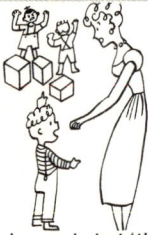

Growing verbal ability. Sometimes expressed in such ways as quarreling, tattling.

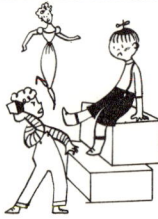

Play still needs some supervision. Quarrels may lead to too much hitting, kicking, throwing.

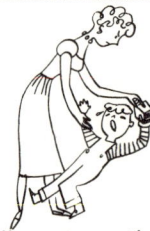

Verbally—and sometimes physically—child dissents from his mother's authority.

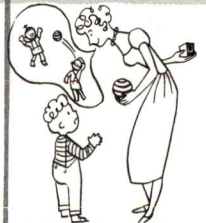

He is beginning to understand rules and restrictions such as balls for throwing—not blocks.

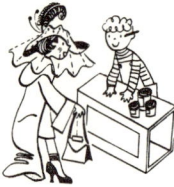

Vivid imagination is frequently expressed in dramatic play, imitation of adults.

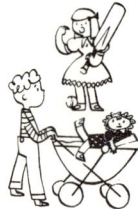

Boys may play with dolls, girls with boyish toys. All right if each enjoys his own toys, too.

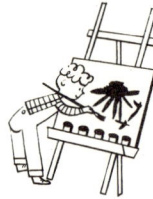

Works hard at drawing—though he may change theme in middle. Details are crude.

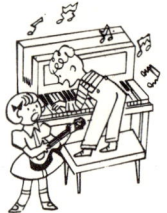

Likes to try musical instruments, play phonograph. Takes part in singing games.

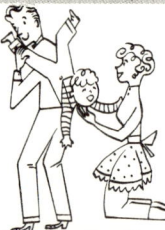

Child frequently clings affectionately to parents. Likes to be cuddled. Enjoys tumbling.

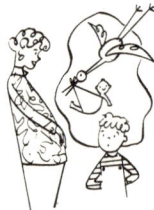

May confuse parents' answers about how babies are born with stories picked up elsewhere.

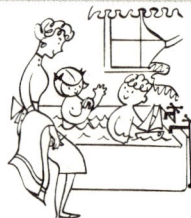

Bathing, toileting of both sexes together offer healthy ways to teach sex differences.

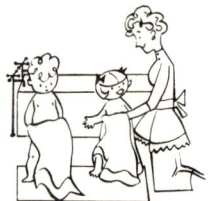

Can bathe himself if mother supervises. Can also partially dry himself.

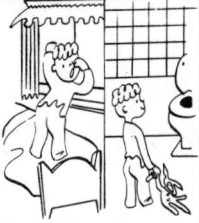

Generally wakes in morning in cheerful humor. Takes care of own immediate needs.

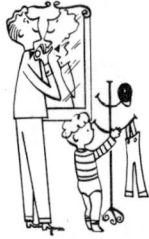

Can almost completely dress himself if clothes are ready at hand.

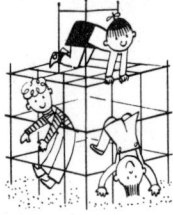

Very energetic. Adept on tricycle and climbing apparatus. Can handle some simple tools.

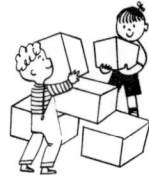

Enjoys nursery school or a play group, since he usually prefers play with others to solitary play.

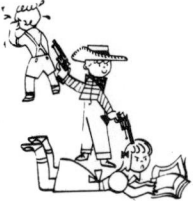

Frequently annoys older brothers and sisters, bullies younger ones.

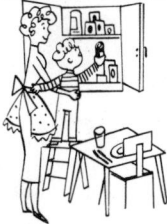

Appetite is fair but improving. Has definite likes and dislikes. Eats skillfully.

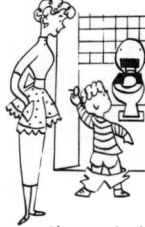

Frequently wants toilet privacy but asks for help with wiping. Controls urination.

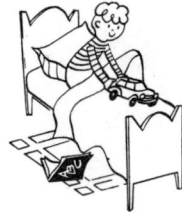

Will rest after lunch, but seldom naps. Plays quietly with books, toys.

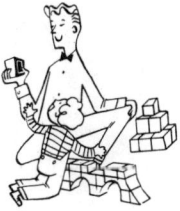

Makes intricate buildings with blocks. Admires his own work. Likes to have father help.

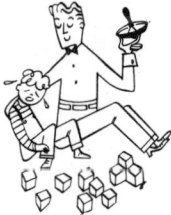

A peak age for crying and whining if bored or hurt. Needs comforting, then distraction.

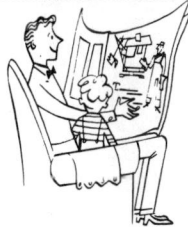

Listens with interest to verse and action stories —especially those explaining how things work.

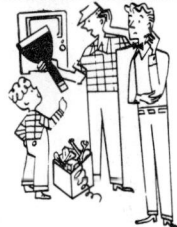

Child is continually asking questions—both to get information and to make conversation.

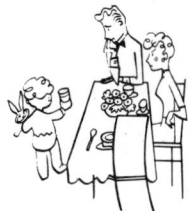

Enjoys eating with family. But interrupts progress of meal by talking, leaving table.

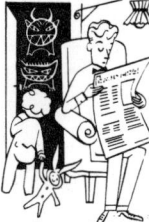

Shows fear of dark, animals, fire engines, old people. May resent mother's going out.

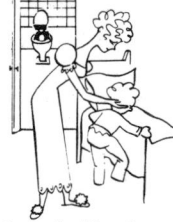

Goes to bed without serious objections— especially if he can recognize bedtime on clock.

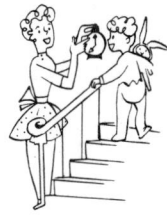

Less awakening because of nightmares now. May wake to go to toilet, needs help getting back.

419

the very special
needs of the child
FROM 5 TO 7

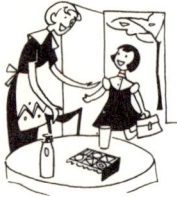

Needs a warm welcome and a chance to talk after a day at school.

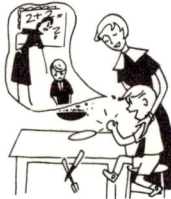

Needs understanding if he occasionally blows his top after a long day of school routine.

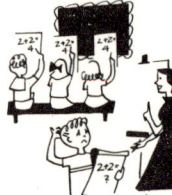

School can give him a feeling of accomplishment, even though he's slow in some things.

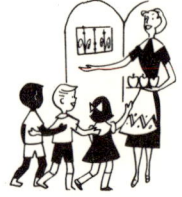

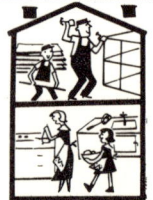

Needs to feel he can freely bring friends home and have parents accept them.

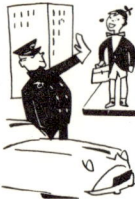

Should be able to take direction but . . .

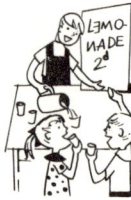

Also needs opportunities to act independently.

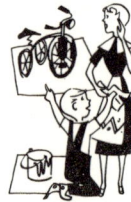

Parents should help with big projects when a child bites off more than he can chew.

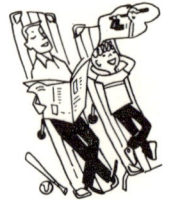

Give him time to think and dream as well as act.

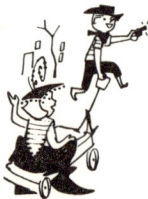

Needs to have opportunity for dressing up and dramatic play.

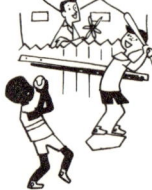

Will easily accept people from other races and groups if parents do not pass on prejudices.

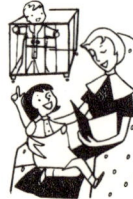

School can give him a feeling of accomplishment, even though he's slow in some things.

Boys need encouragement to develop masculine traits, girls to develop feminine ones.

What your school beginner needs at this crucial time when he is entering a big new world. A feature based on scientific studies

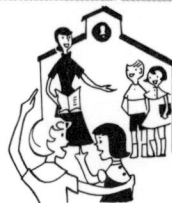

Make him feel that starting school is an adventure, not banishment to a disciplinary place.

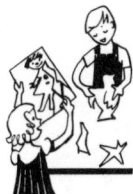

Give him opportunities for creative activity adapted to his own capacities.

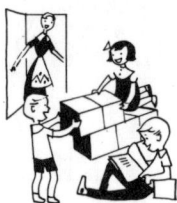

Parents can help by realizing that he will learn to read when he's ready, not at a special age.

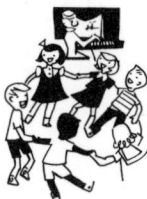

He needs simple spontaneous group play and skipping, dancing, rhythmic activity.

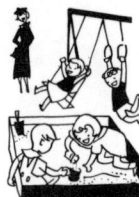

Needs space and materials for play—from which he learns much.

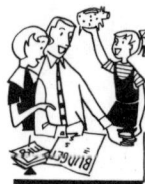

Needs an allowance to develop a sense of the value of money.

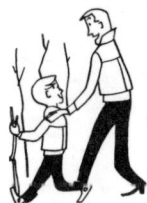

Parent of the same sex as child should make opportunities for companionship.

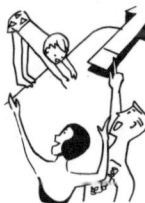

Build him up by emphasizing his strong points, rather than criticizing his weaknesses.

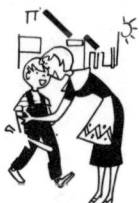

Is mature enough to spend time away from home but still needs assurance of parents' love.

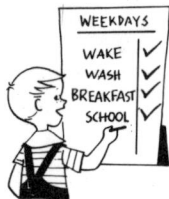

Needs the comfort of a regular but flexible routine.

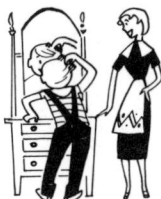

Start his training in habits of personal hygiene but . . .

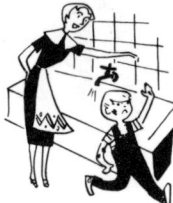

Try to be tolerant toward rowdiness and personal sloppiness characteristic of his age.

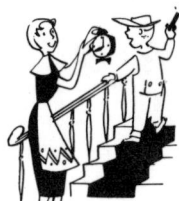

Needs about 11 hours of sleep every night.

421

meeting the needs of the child
FROM 8 TO 10

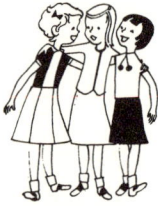

Needs to feel accepted and approved by his own age group—dislikes being alone.

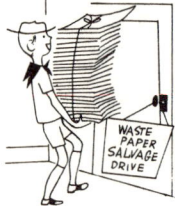

Enjoys feeling important and useful. Likes club activities, Scouting.

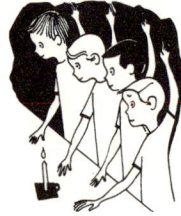

Relishes the tribal excitement of membership in a tight and secret group.

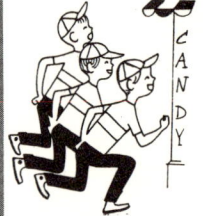

Conforms to his gang's standards of dress, speech, games and manners.

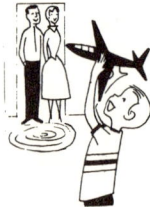

Looks for the reassurance of parents' understanding and support.

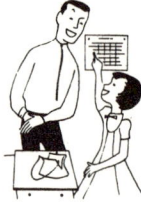

Allowance or earnings helps him learn value of money, independence.

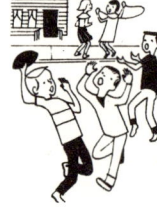

Running, jumping, other strenuous, hard-on-adults activities are necessary.

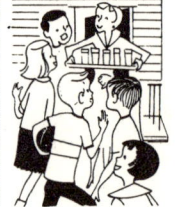

But adults must be watchful to forestall exhaustion or overstimulation.

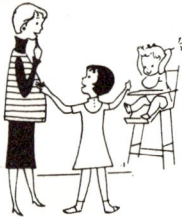

Parents who answer sex questions frankly are helpful.

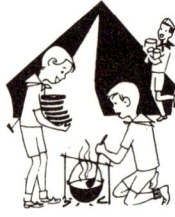

Activities away from home give scope to his yen for adventure.

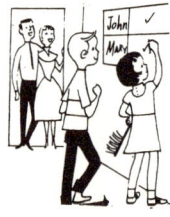

Helping with household tasks gets him used to shouldering obligations.

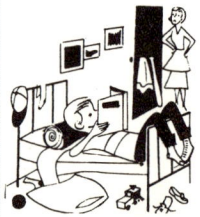

Needs realization by parents that he's not yet ready for adult conduct.

Less home centered, more social minded,
your child meets new responsibilities
in these years. Here's a cross section
of research on his special needs

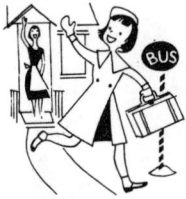

Wants freedom
to visit alone
and to play host to
friends at home.

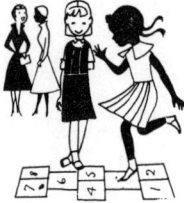

Needs adult
example and
guidance on tolerance,
morals, life goals.

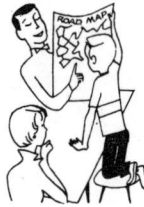

Likes to par-
ticipate in
family planning
and activity.

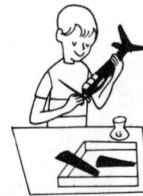

Needs satisfac-
tion of starting
projects,
completing them.

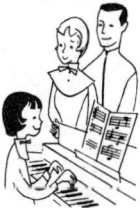

Must know that
parents are
sympathetic to his
creative interests.

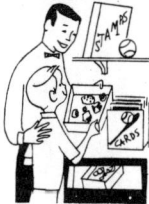

Needs patience
with his rash of
special and usually
short-term interests.

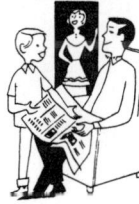

Broadens mentally
with practice
in discussion,
arguments, reasoning.

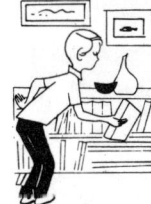

Has to develop his
own taste in
literature. Needs good
books readily available.

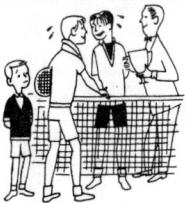

Unobtrusive aid
helps him to develop
his own standards
of decency, fair play.

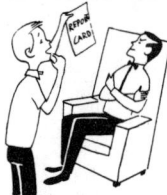

Needs tolerance of
his nervous gestures
—and a parental review
as to their source.

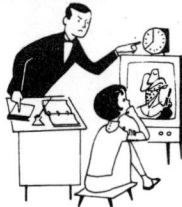

Should have an
agreement with
parents about time for
homework, TV, movies.

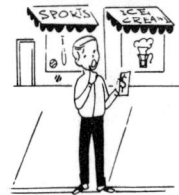

Matures when allowed
to make decisions and
face non-serious
consequences of mistake.

prime needs of
11-13 YEAR OLDS

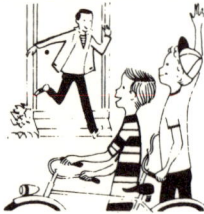

They need to feel accepted by their age group and to take an active role within it.

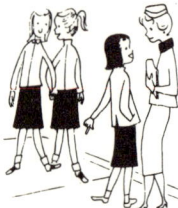

Want to conform to group's standards for dress, activities, possessions.

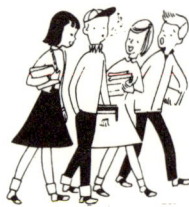

Begin to develop friendships with opposite sex and need to feel at ease with them.

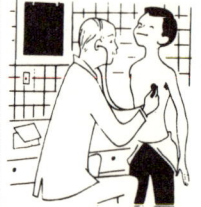

An understanding of his own body, its changes and its capacities is important.

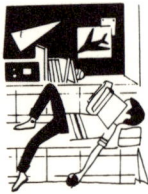

Appreciates moments of privacy and—if possible —a room of his own.

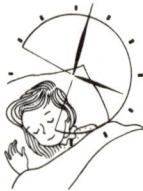

Generally needs eight to ten hours of sleep a night.

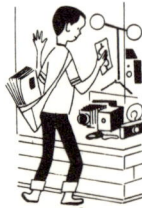

Wants enough money from odd jobs and his allowance to finance his personal projects.

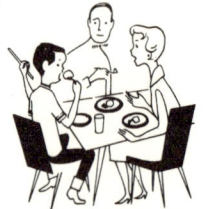

Looks to adults for guidance as to what is considered good manners and behavior.

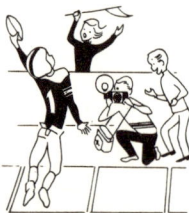

Thrive when they shine in some activity admired by their group.

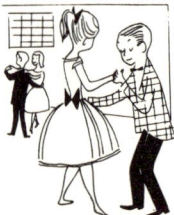

Welcome opportunity to learn social dancing —though boys may be reluctant to admit this.

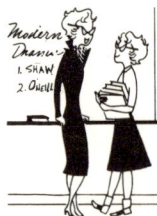

Should be spoken to and directed on the basis of mutual respect.

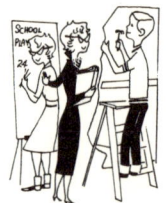

Chooses some admired adult for her model of dignity and good sense.

*Conformity to the group, independence
toward parents, mark this as an important
self-testing period. But tactful
guidance is welcome*

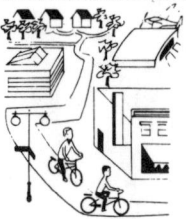

Should have chance to broaden their first-hand experience with the world around them.

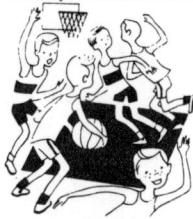

Like to play games which require high degree of teamwork and organization.

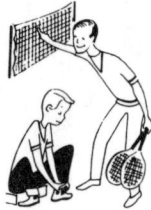

They should be encouraged to try their skill with new sports.

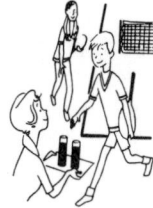

Require supervision to make sure they don't get too tired from strenuous play.

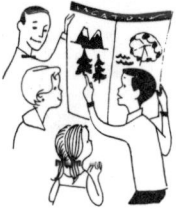

Wants to feel that his views play an important role in family discussions.

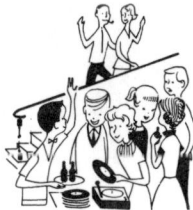

Must have the freedom to organize social activities on grown-up lines.

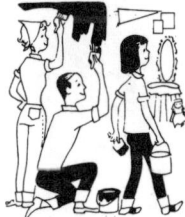

Gains family status by being given family responsibilities within her capabilities.

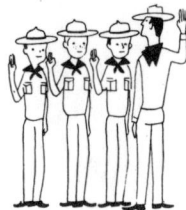

Need the goal of a high minded moral code such as religion, Boy Scouts.

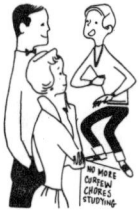

Needs tolerance toward his revolt against adult ways and standards.

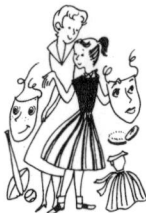

Assurance and guidance foster a positive attitude toward sex roles.

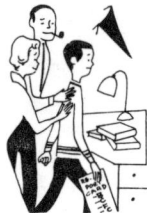

Parents' open recognition that he is a worthwhile individual is essential.

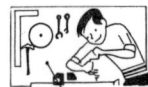

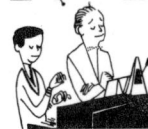

Careful attention must be paid to development of individual potentialities.

14 TO 16
are crucial years in growing up

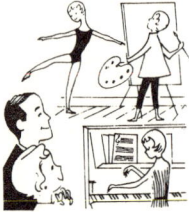
Needs active encouragement for steadily broadening intellectual and aesthetic interests.

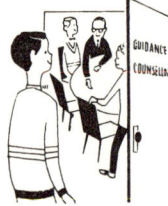
Should have expert counsel on his future course toward a vocation or higher education.

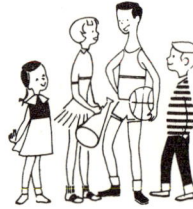
Wants a chance to excel in sports or some other activity.

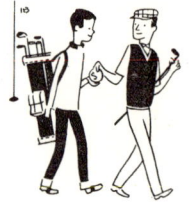
Needs chances to earn money and decide how to use his own earnings.

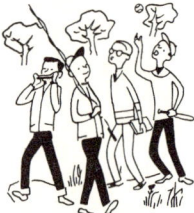
Requires freedom to choose leisure time activities and to enjoy them in his own way.

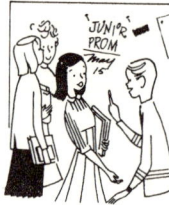
Needs confidence in his attractiveness for the opposite sex.

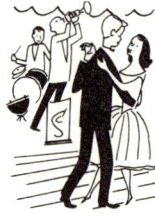
Appreciates instruction in and opportunity for social contacts with opposite sex.

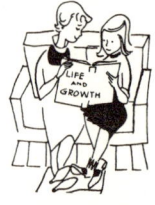
Must have factual knowledge about sex and reassurance that feelings are not to be feared.

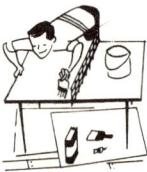
Must be made responsible for personal possessions and hobby equipment.

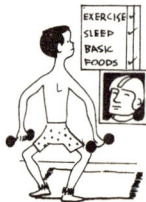
Should be encouraged to accept responsibility for his own health and general well being.

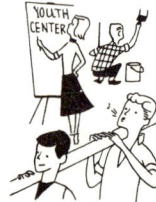
Looks for worthy projects on which to expend abundant physical and emotional energy.

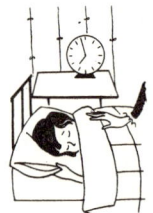
As a rule requires 8-10 hours sleep a night.

*Mid-teens is a training ground for
responsible adulthood. Understanding
parents will alternate their helping hand
with a hands-off policy*

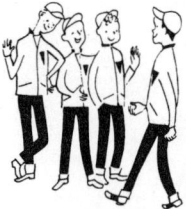

Acceptance and approval by his gang are very important to him.

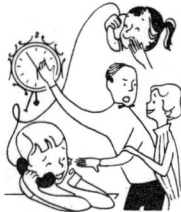

Needs the freedom to develop deep friendships.

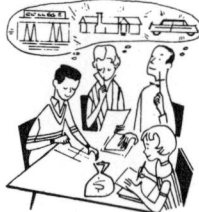

Appreciates opportunity to share in family planning and family responsibilities.

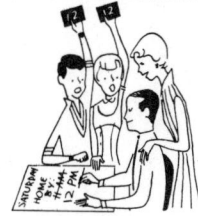

Wants a part in making decisions as to the degree of freedom which he may have.

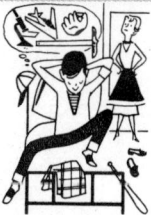

Asks for tolerance through those long inactive periods of the "figuring things out process."

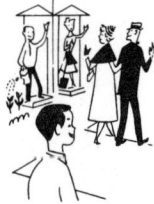

Wants his parents to be models of appropriate behavior.

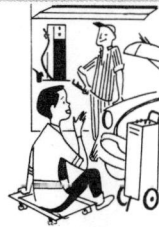

Must have friendships with adults other than his parents to gain insight into other points of view.

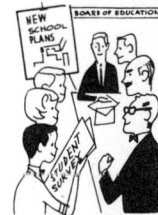

Wants encouragement and goals in his growing awareness of social and community problems.

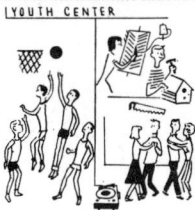

After-school and holiday youth center program foster interests, curb delinquency.

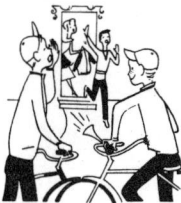

Tolerant attitude toward his need to be rough, tough and noisy is essential.

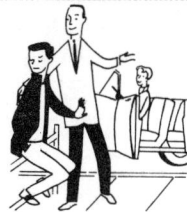

Especially needs parents' realization that his aggressiveness and rejection of them are only temporary.

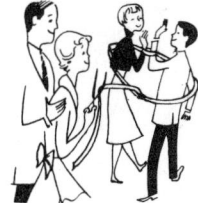

Thrives on family relationship which balances understanding, affection, freedom.

EXPECTED INCREASES IN WEIGHTS AND HEIGHTS

(from infancy to the teens)

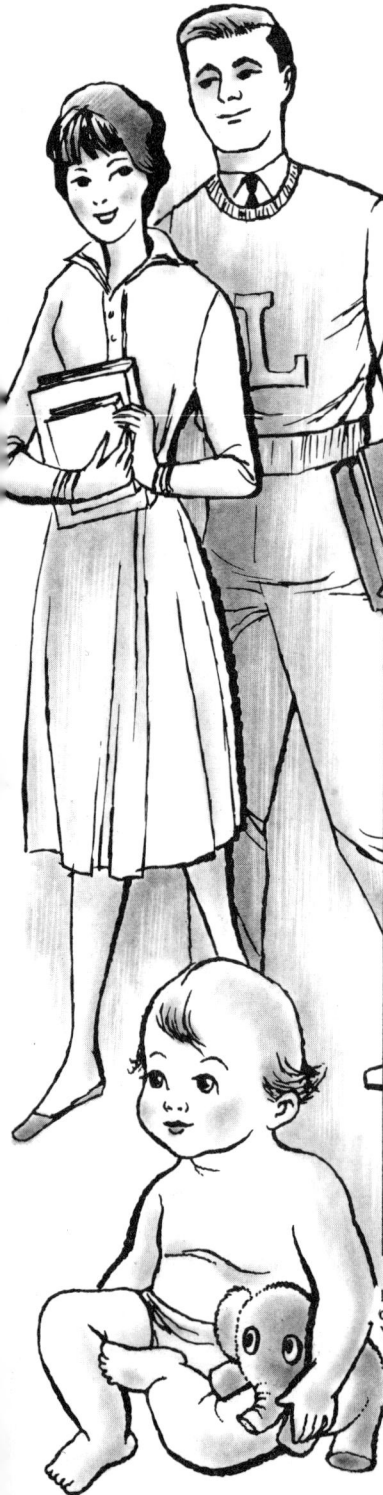

AGE	BOYS AND GIRLS WEIGHT IN POUNDS		BOYS AND GIRLS HEIGHT IN INCHES	
0-1 mo.	1.4		1.5	
1-3 mo.	3.4		2.4	
3-6 mo.	3.9		2.5	
6-9 mo.	3.0		1.8	
9-12 mo.	2.2		1.6	
12-18 mo.	3.1		2.6	
18-24 mo.	2.7		2.2	
24-30 mo.	2.3		1.9	
30-36 mo.	2.1		1.7	
36-42 mo.	2.3		1.5	
42-48 mo.	2.1		1.4	
48-54 mo.	2.4		1.4	
54-60 mo.	2.2		1.3	
60-66 mo.	2.5		1.4	
66-72 mo.	2.6		1.3	
	BOYS	GIRLS	BOYS	GIRLS
6-7 yr.	4.9	4.6	2.4	2.3
7-8 yr.	5.2	4.9	2.2	2.2
8-9 yr.	5.5	5.6	2.2	2.2
9-10 yr.	5.9	6.1	2.0	2.1
10-11 yr.	5.5	7.6	2.0	2.3
11-12 yr.	6.5	9.9	2.0	2.5
12-13 yr.	9.0	11.3	2.2	2.6
13-14 yr.	12.0	9.5	3.6	2.0
14-15 yr.	11.3	5.0	2.3	1.0
15-16 yr.	9.8	4.0	2.0	0.8
16-17 yr.	7.0	2.6	1.5	0.3

Data from "Growth and Development
of Children," Watson and Lowrey,
Year Book Publishers

CHILL, a sensation of cold, accompanied by shivering and usually with teeth chattering, throbbing, and trembling. It is frequently a prominent early symptom of acute infection. Any severe chill during a fever is a danger signal and a doctor should be called at once.

A chill results from an increase in the chemical activity going on in the body and therefore a rapid rise in the production of heat by the body. The ultimate result of a chill is increased body temperature. A person with a chill is usually quiet, lies doubled up, has a pale cool skin and sometimes "goose flesh," due to the constriction of the superficial blood vessels under the skin which is sometimes so great that the skin appears blue. A mild chill can usually be controlled to some degree by the person; however, a severe chill cannot. Warm blankets and clothing, hot drinks, hot-water bottles, and electric pads will help relieve the discomfort of the person with chills.

A chill can be induced in patients by injecting certain nonspecific protein substances. It can also be prevented by drugs which act as sedatives and as controls of body temperature. The action of these drugs, which are known as antipyretic and antifever drugs, is to depress the activity of the center in the brain which controls chills and shivering.

The chill is being studied to gain further knowledge as to its cause and significance. Many physicians feel that a chill is often of real importance in helping to overcome a disease since it raises the body temperature through muscular movement. *See also* FEVER.

CHILL — brass: See article OCCUPATION AND HEALTH, page 1385.

CHILL — scarlet fever: See article INFECTIOUS DISEASES OF CHILDHOOD, page 1112-13.

CHILL — zinc: See article OCCUPATION AND HEALTH, page 1385.

CHIROPRACTIC, a therapeutic system based on the theory that the bones of the spinal column, by pressing on the spinal nerves, cause an interruption of the normal function of the nerves. The result of this pressure is said to be eventual damage to the tissues. Extensive medical investigation has failed to show any scientific foundation for this system. Chiropractors are nevertheless licensed to practice in most states. Practically all chiropractors are in the United States.

CHLOASMA. *See* LIVER SPOTS.

CHLOROFORM, trichloromethane, a heavy colorless liquid with a typical ether smell. Chloroform is best known as an anesthetic, and has been used for that purpose since 1847 when Dr. James Simpson, an Edinburgh gynecologist, dissatisfied with ether, discovered the narcotic qualities of chloroform. It became fashionable as an anesthetic in childbirth when Queen Victoria permitted its administration during the delivery of her seventh child.

Too large quantities and habitual use of chloroform may result in poisoning, injuries to the liver and kidneys, a condition of transient albuminuria, albumin present in the urine, and other diseases. *See also* ANESTHESIA.

CHLOROFORM — albuminuria may result: See article THE KIDNEY: ITS DISEASES AND DISTURBANCES, page 1177.

CHLOROFORM — industrial poison: See article OCCUPATION AND HEALTH, page 1377.

CHLOROFORM — liver injured: See article DIGESTION AND DIGESTIVE DISEASES, page 891.

CHLOROFORM — nephrosis: See article THE KIDNEY: ITS DISEASES AND DISTURBANCES, page 1193.

CHLOROFORM—poisoning: See article FIRST AID, page 829.

CHLOROSIS, a form of anemia, characterized by a large reduction of hemoglobin in the blood, but with only a slight diminution in the number of red cells. Some decades ago, chlorosis, or "green sickness," was common among girls and young women, but today it has almost completely disappeared because of increased knowledge of the place of iron in the diet. The symptoms of this iron deficiency are a greenish color to the skin, and menstrual and gastric disturbances.

CHOLECYSTITIS, the scientific name for inflammation of the gallbladder. *See also* GALLBLADDER.

CHOLECYSTITIS — See article DIGESTION AND DIGESTIVE DISTURBANCES, page 888.

CHOLECYSTOGRAPHY, roentgenography, x-ray diagnosis, of the gallbladder after it has been made visual by substances not transparent to the x-ray.

Gallstone attacks have characteristic symptoms, yet differences in related symptoms and severity of pain often makes a definite distinction from other diseases difficult. The introduction of cholecystography has been a great advance in the diagnosis of gallstones.

CHOLELITHIASIS, a condition associated with calculi, stones in the gallbladder or in a bile duct. *See also* GALLBLADDER.

CHOLERA, an acute infection which chiefly involves the small intestine. The main symptoms are severe, constantly flowing diarrhea, vomiting, collapse, cramps in the muscles, and suppression of the flow of urine from the kidneys.

Cholera spreads most rapidly in moist warm climates. From time immemorial it has existed in India, from where at one time it spread throughout the world, probably traveling along caravan routes into Europe and along water trade routes.

The cause of cholera was described some fifty years ago by the German researcher, Robert Koch. A germ, the comma bacillus, gains entrance into the body through polluted drinking water. The organism then gets into the bowel where it causes acute infection. Cholera spreads in much the same way as typhoid fever does, the germs escaping from the body along with material that is vomited or passed from the bowel.

To prevent the spread of cholera, the cholera patient must be isolated. Material that is passed from the patient must be destroyed by fire. Only food that has been cooked, and boiled, or preferably chlorinated, water should be used by people in an area where cholera exists. The food and water should not be permitted to stand for any length of time since they may become recontaminated. Those who live or travel in cholera-ridden areas can be partially protected against this disease through vaccination with a serum made from the killed bodies of the specific cholera germs. The incidence of cholera among inoculated people has been low.

About five or six days after a person has been infected with cholera, a severe diarrhea begins, with violent purging, and eventually practically pure mucus and water are passed. Then vomiting begins, followed by collapse. The skin loses its elasticity, the muscles cramp, the eyes are sunken, and the voice is feeble. As more and more water is lost, the thirst becomes intense, the pulse becomes rapid and weak, and the blood pressure falls. The face becomes sunken and the skin develops a blue, cyanotic tinge, as the blood gradually loses its oxygen. As the patient's condition improves, the reverse of the process occurs.

Whenever large amounts of fluid are lost from the body, danger of death from acid intoxication ensues. Therefore, the chief step in the treatment is restoration of the fluid. Large quantities of normal or physiological salt solution are given to the patient by injection into the veins. Delay may be fatal, and frequently it is necessary to give one or two quarts of this solution, every six or eight hours, for two or three days. The acidosis may be overcome by giving large doses of sodium bicarbonate. Usually the person with cholera is content to remain in bed.

Warmth is sustained by blankets, hot-water bottles, and electric pads. The physician can help to control the vomiting by prescription of proper remedies.

In the United States, cholera has ceased to be a serious problem, although it still occurs in many other parts of the world.

CHOLERA — cause determined: See article THE PREVENTION AND TREATMENT OF INFECTIOUS DISEASE, page 1090.
CHOLERA — incidence: See article THE PREVENTION AND TREATMENT OF INFECTIOUS DISEASE, page 1095-96.
CHOLERA — infected water most common source: See article DIGESTION AND DIGESTIVE DISEASES, page 897.

CHOLESTEROL, a fatty substance, a basis for hundreds of chemical processes in the body. Animal meat, cream, butter, and eggs contain large amounts of cholesterol and its presence in excess amounts in the blood stream is believed by many medical investigators to be responsible for a type of arterial hardening known as atherosclerosis. In this disease, cholesterol plaques in the inside wall of arteries cause the wall to thicken and roughen. Ultimately the flow of blood through that portion of the artery is restricted, or a piece of the roughened wall may tear away and block the flow of blood to those tissues served by the artery. When this occurs in the arteries that supply the heart muscle with blood the condition is called coronary thrombosis.

Dr. John Gofman and his associates at the University of California have proposed that a definite correlation exists between severe coronary heart attacks and excess blood cholesterol. Other medical investigators have produced atherosclerosis in animals by feeding them diets high in cholesterol. Certain heart specialists advocate a low-fat, low-cholesterol diet to prevent or control coronary heart disease, but others believe that since the body produces its own cholesterol, dietary restriction of it will not help appreciably. Investigations indicate that factors other than the existence of excess cholesterol may be responsible for arterial hardening. These may involve the body's ability to metabolize the cholesterol, or its ratio to other substances, such as protein and phosphatides, in the blood stream, the size and number of the cholesterol molecules, and the effect of exercise on the amount of circulating cholesterol. In one experiment, Dr. Frederick J. Stare of Harvard University's School of Public Health reports a definite correlation between exercise and a reduction in certain types of cholesterol molecules.

CHOLESTEROL — arteriosclerosis may be developed by: See article DIABETES, page 578-79.

CHOLESTEROL — gallstones: See article DIGESTION AND DIGESTIVE DISEASES, page 888.

CHONDROMA, a slowly developing tumor growing from tissues or cartilage. In the chest this tumor tends to spread toward important organs. Generally benign, chondroma may recur after removal by surgery.

CHOREA, more familiarly known as St. Vitus' dance, a disease of the nervous system which causes involuntary twitching of various parts of the body. Children prior to puberty are most often affected.

Unlike many diseases of the nervous system, St. Vitus' dance normally lasts a relatively short time, often no more than twelve weeks. Sometimes relapses occur, and in other instances the disease may endure for one or two years, although not usually.

Chorea is believed to be the result of a general streptococcus infection which in some apparently indirect way, perhaps through toxic substances developed by the germs of the infection, strikes at the brain and the nervous system. Children may develop a temporary, habitual twitch from imitating the movements of other people, but this is completely different in origin and in character from the involuntary twitching that is seen in St. Vitus' dance.

The onset of the disease, which often accompanies rheumatic fever, may appear as a generalized illness with fever, vomiting, and headache, along with dizziness and weakness. The first disturbances of bodily movement are often mistaken for clumsiness of the child. However, the true nature of the ailment soon becomes apparent.

When fully developed, the movements are rapid, of short duration, and distinctive; none exactly duplicates any that preceded. Muscular coordination becomes difficult and approximately 25 per cent of the cases are so severe as to disturb the speech function. The child becomes irritable and restless, and his memory, attention span, and emotions may be mildly disturbed.

The treatment of chorea, a disease implicating the whole system and not just isolated parts, begins with prolonged bed rest of three to six weeks at least. Because of the close relationship to streptococcus infection, the child should be kept under close observation. Any infection of the throat, in the tonsils or adenoids, in the teeth or elsewhere should be eliminated quickly and the child kept in bed. Both in streptococcus infections and in chorea attention must be given the heart, which may be particularly affected. The use of penicillin or sulfa is recommended by the American Heart Association to prevent streptococcal infection and to protect against a recurrence of rheumatic fever.

Baths and sedative drugs directed at alleviating the symptoms of chorea are frequently quite helpful. Both heat and drugs striking at the infection itself are often beneficial, but neither are specifically effective.

Convalescence of the patient with chorea should be gradual, with a nutritional diet assuring plenty of vitamins and minerals. Exercise and play should be resumed in moderation and under supervision, but the child must relax and not overdo. *See also* ATAXIA.

CHOREA—See article DISEASES OF THE HEART AND CIRCULATION, pages 990, 992.

CHORION, the outermost of the fetal membranes which covers, nourishes, and protects the developing ovum. Later it becomes the fetal part of the placenta.

CHROMOBLASTOMYCOSIS, a rare skin infection caused by a fungus which grows on plants and trees in warm humid areas. Only a few cases have been reported in the United States, but the disease occurs more frequently in South America.

The infection usually starts on the feet or legs. The skin turns purplish red and develops colored, warty, cauliflower-like growths. X-ray, used externally in combination with appropriate drugs, has successfully disposed of the fungus and the growths. A potential danger, however, in any such disorder is that the offending organism will reach the lung or some other vital part where it may cause death.

CHRONIC signifies long-continued or of long duration. A chronic disease is prolonged, often slowly progressing and never completely cured —as, for example, chronic bronchitis or chronic arthritis.

CHRONIC – chronic disorders reduce resistance to other diseases: See article THE PREVENTION AND TREATMENT OF INFECTIOUS DISEASE, page 1092-94.

CHRYSAROBIN, an orange powder, derived from the bark of a Brazilian tree, which stains the skin a deep brown. It is used to treat psoriasis, and is also effective in fungus infections called dhobie itch and gym or jockey itch, involving the skin of the groin, perineum, and perianal regions.

CHRYSAROBIN – See article THE SKIN, page 1776.

CILIA, fine, hairlike appendages which cover the surface of mucous membranes, the moist sensitive lining of the respiratory tract. The cilia are filtering organisms, a protective measure to keep harmful particles out of the lung. They move upward and downward, and through the more pronounced upward movement, mucus, dust, and other infectious particles are swept and propelled toward the mouth, so that they are not breathed into the lungs. Eyelashes are also cilia, and protect the eyes from foreign particles.

CIRCULATORY SYSTEM. The heart pumps the blood through a "pipeline" of closed tubes or vessels. This pipeline forms two major circular routes in the body, the systemic circulation and the pulmonary circulation, with the heart acting as a central pump. The circulatory system, with its major and minor routes, reaches every cell in the body, bringing the blood with its life-sustaining products from the organs where they are manufactured to the tissues where they are needed. It also carries away the waste products to other organs in the body, where they are broken down and either converted to be used again or excreted as waste. In addition, the circulatory system takes care of the more active organs by bringing them an increased flow of blood, whereas those organs which are less active, or temporarily at rest, receive less blood.

The heart is divided into a right side and a left side. Each side is further divided into two chambers an auricle and a ventricle. The auricles are the collecting depots for the blood, while the ventricles pump the blood out of the heart into the blood vessels.

In the systemic circulation, the blood is pumped from the left ventricle into the aorta, or large artery, passing through a series of smaller arteries which branch from it, then continues through the arterioles, or smallest arteries, which end in a fine network of tiny vessels called the capillaries. The capillaries transfer the blood, with its oxygen and nutriment, to the various tissues of the body and then conduct it from the tissues into the venules, or tiny veins, on through larger veins until it finally reaches the inferior vena cava, one of the two great veins on the right side of the heart. From here, it passes into the right auricle, and thus completes the systemic circle. The blood, venous blood, dark in color, which enters the right auricle, has deposited most of its oxygen, and has picked the carbon dioxide from the tissues.

Before the blood can resume its systemic flow, it must secure a fresh supply of oxygen. The right ventricle now pumps the blood through the pulmonary artery into the capillaries of the lungs, where it deposits its carbon dioxide and gathers up the new oxygen. This blood, now a bright red, is arterial blood which then enters the pulmonary vein, flows into the left auricle from which it enters the left ventricle, and is then ready to start on its route through the body again. This circuitous routine is the pulmonary circulation.

In addition to these two major circulations, some of the blood stream from the systemic circulation is diverted by the capillaries of the stomach and intestinal tract to the portal

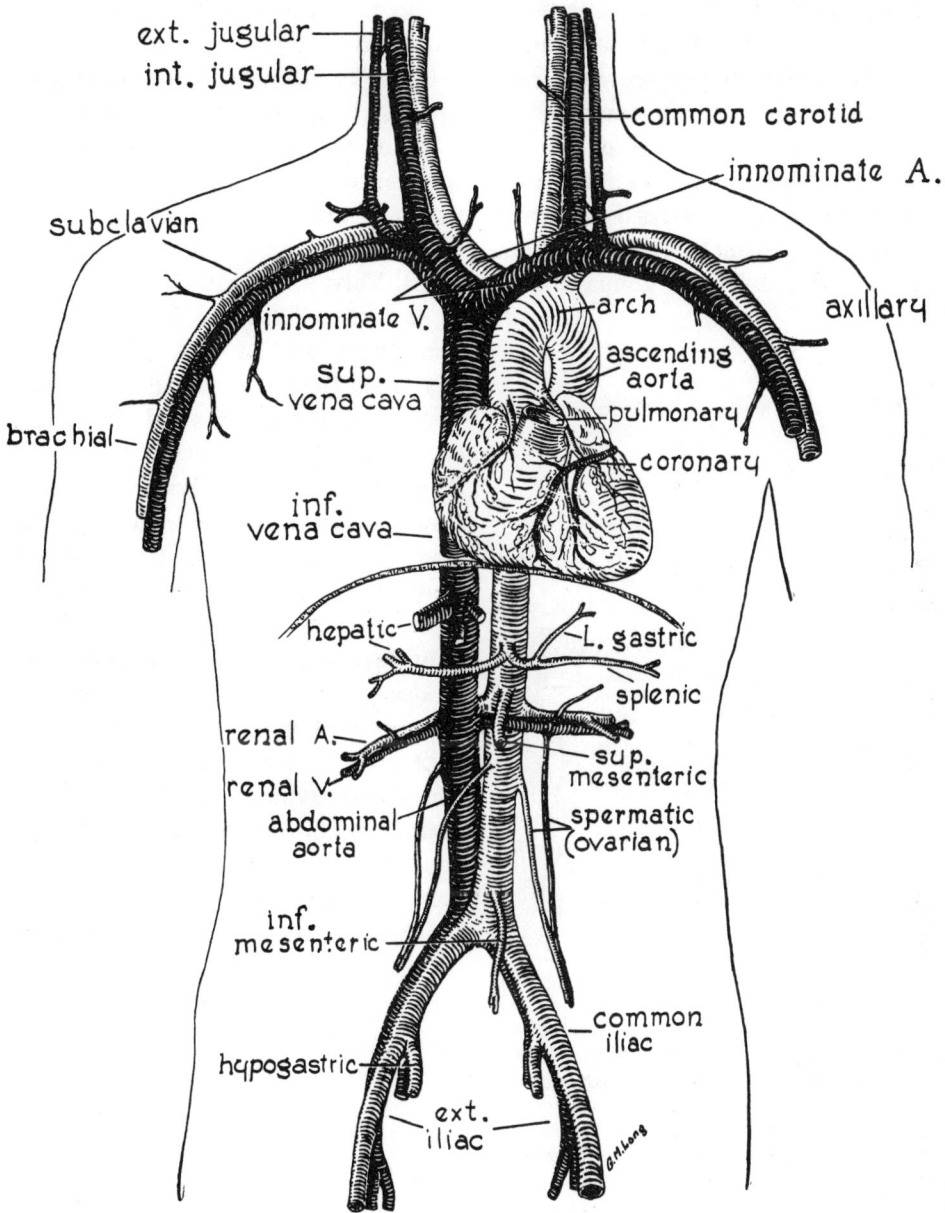

Circulatory System—The veins and arteries of the human torso. The veins are the darker vessels. Blood circulates from the aorta to the arteries and then to the smaller arteries, returning to the heart (the sac-like structure) by way of the veins.

vein and is carried to the liver, which acts as a storage depot for blood. Here some of the impurities are removed and excreted into the digestive tract, and the blood is returned through the hepatic vein to the superior vena cava of the heart. This system is the portal circulation. Another accessory circulation from the systemic feeds blood to the kidneys

435

and is called the renal circulation. The coronary arteries, veins, and their capillaries supply the heart itself with oxygen and nutriments and remove waste material, and constitute the coronary circulation. The brain and head are served by the two carotid arteries which bring the blood supply, and also by the jugular veins

which carry away the blood and waste materials.

The circulatory pipeline consists of the three types of blood vessels described: the arteries, the veins, and the capillaries. The capillaries connect the ends of the smallest arteries to the beginnings of the smallest veins. Valves inside the heart and also in the veins keep the flow of blood continuous and in one direction. In the veins they are spaced at various distances, opening toward the heart, so that the flow cannot go backward. The valves control the rate of the flow and its distribution through the body. The final control of the blood flow is exerted by the capillaries, which are so small that the blood cells can pass through only in single or double file.

The walls of the capillaries are a thin layer of fine platelike cells, endothelium, which are dovetailed to form a membranous network where the blood deposits its nutriment, oxygen, and other substances needed by the body tissues, and from which it

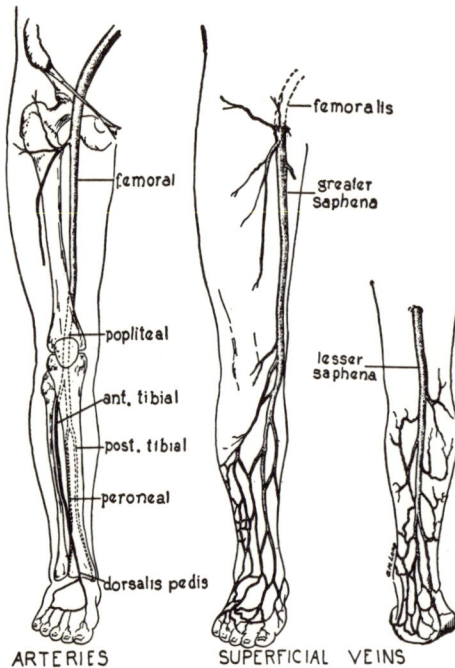

Circulatory System—The arteries and veins of the leg and thigh. The large artery of the thigh is the femoral *(left)*, while the large vein of the lower extremity is the long saphenous vein, or saphena. This vein begins on the inner side of the foot *(right)* and extends up the inside of the leg and thigh, joining the femoral vein, or femoralis, in the groin *(center)*.

Circulatory System—The arteries and veins of the arm and hand. The axillary, the large artery of the arm *(left)*, divides into the ulnar and radial arteries. The radial artery at the wrist is the one used in taking the pulse.

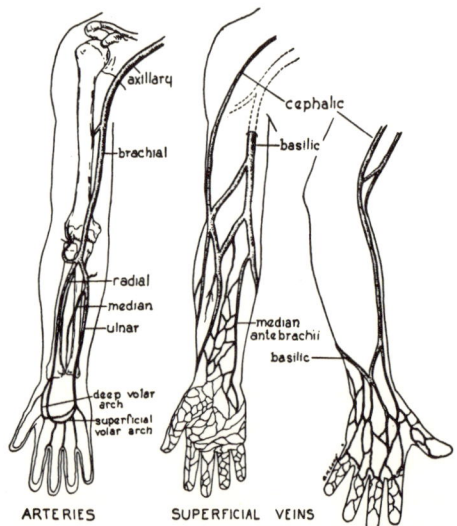

THE PATH OF BLOOD THROUGH THE HEART

GREAT VEIN FROM HEAD AND ARMS

ARTERY FROM RIGHT HEART TO LUNGS

GREAT ARTERY FROM LEFT HEART TO BODY

VEIN FROM RIGHT LUNG TO LEFT HEART

VEIN FROM LEFT LUNG TO LEFT HEART

GREAT VEIN FROM BODY AND LEGS

RIGHT HEART

LEFT HEART

Chart by GRAPHICS INSTITUTE

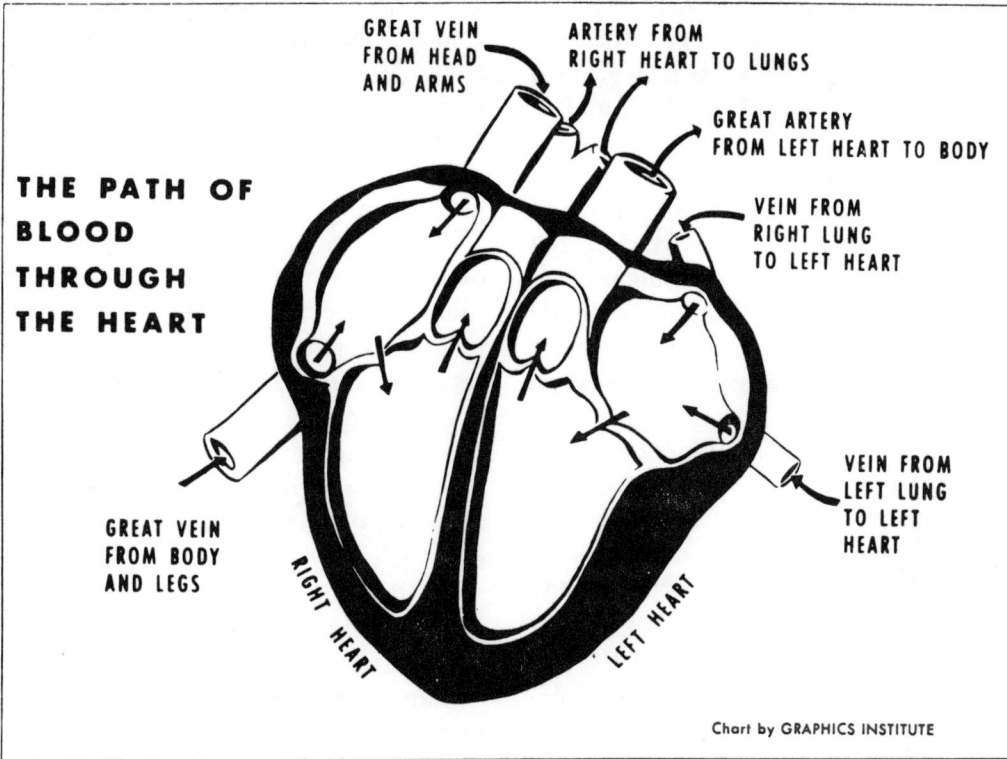

Circulatory System — Chart shows the path of blood through the heart as it comes in by the veins and goes out through arteries. Large veins bring the blood into the right heart, then arteries conduct blood from the right heart to the lungs. Blood from the lungs goes to the left heart through veins and goes out of the left heart to the body through the great artery (aorta).

picks up the gases and other waste products. Those tissues which are not reached easily by this interchange receive their nutriment from the liquid constituents of the blood, which also filter through the capillary network and carry food and oxygen to the tissues. This clear fluid which filters out of the capillaries is the tissue fluid. The capillaries are found throughout all tissues and organs of the body, and are more numerous, where the body organs are most active. Over a million capillaries may run through a square inch of muscle

tissue, and if all the capillaries were joined in a single tube it would stretch for thousands of miles.

The walls of the arteries must be thick and strong to accommodate the stream of blood within them which is pumped by the heart under great pressure. They consist of three layers, the endothelium, or fine inner layer; the middle layer, on which the strength and caliber of the vessel depends, which is a thick coat of strong muscle fibers and heavy elastic tissue permitting expansion and contraction of the artery; and the outside coat, or adventitia, a thick layer of connective tissue which gives the vessel elasticity and enables it to act as a reservoir for the blood flow, and at the same time prevents the blood from oozing into the tissues.

The walls of the veins are structurally similar to the arteries, but they are thinner and their diameter is much larger since the flow of blood through the veins and into the heart is under less pressure and slower in rate.

In the course of normal routine, and more so in disease, much strain is placed upon the structures that constitute the circulatory system. As cells deteriorate, new cells replace them. Fortunately not all the cells wear out at the same time, and the process of replacement continues throughout life, so that a steady balance is maintained between the removal of worn-out cells by the circulating blood and the regeneration of new cells. *See also* CORONARY THROMBOSIS; EMBOLISM; HEART; LYMPHATIC SYSTEM.

CIRCULATORY SYSTEM — arthritis may result from disturbances: See article ARTHRITIS, RHEUMATISM, AND GOUT, page 156-57.

CIRCULATORY SYSTEM — bathing has beneficial effect: See article THE SKIN, page 1728.

CIRCULATORY SYSTEM — contrast bath: See article THE FOOT, page 768.

CIRCULATORY SYSTEM — diseases: See article DISEASES OF THE HEART AND CIRCULATION, page 978-1020.

CIRCULATORY SYSTEM—rheumatism may result from disturbances: See article ARTHRITIS, RHEUMATISM, AND GOUT, page 156-57.

CIRCUMCISION, is the surgical removal of the loose fold of the skin, the foreskin, which covers the head of the penis.

Circumcision was originally a religious rite in ancient Egypt and among Hebrews, Mohammedans, South Sea Islanders, and American Indians. The Book of Genesis interprets circumcision as a blood covenant, and it is still practiced as such among some Jews.

Today the operation is still recommended by many doctors as a routine hygienic measure, or to diminish the possibility of contracting venereal diseases. With improved sanitary conditions, permitting frequent bathing and washing, circumcision as a sanitary measure is probably not as significant as it formerly was.

The best time for the operation is before the infant is ten days old, when it represents a minor procedure. Circumcision should always be done under strictest surgical or aseptic conditions. Proper repair of the tissues after the extra skin has been removed is essential. If the doctor's instructions regarding protection and cleansing of the wound are carefully followed, complications are rare.

Circumcision is recommended when the foreskin is unusually long so that it retains urine which might cause infection. Inflammation and irritation under the foreskin are also associated with various nervous manifestations.

CIRCUMCISION — See article SEX HYGIENE, page 1671-72.

CIRCUMCISION — cancer of penis prevented by: See article CANCER, page 320-21.

CIRCUMCISION—recommended when cleanliness impossible without it: See article SEX HYGIENE, page 1701-02.

CIRCUMCISION—sometimes called for when children pull at genitals: See article SEX HYGIENE, page 1679-80.

CIRRHOSIS, a chronic progressive disease, essentially inflammatory, with a pathological hardening of tissue brought about by an increase of connective tissue elements. The lungs, ovaries, heart, or stomach may be affected with cirrhosis, but it occurs more often in the kidney and liver.

Cirrhosis of the kidney, chronic interstitial nephritis, is a chronic inflammation of the connective tissue elements of the kidney. Cirrhosis of the liver, the most frequent type, is usually a disease of adults but may occasionally occur in younger people, and is three times more common among men than women. It involves a scarring or hardening of the liver, produced by an overgrowth of the connective tissue elements to the neglect of the true hepatic cells.

Heavy consumers of alcohol are often victims of cirrhosis, but moderate drinkers may become affected. The disease may also be caused by bacterial infection, particularly from bacteria of the colon, infectious cirrhosis. *See also* LIVER.

CIRRHOSIS – See article DIGESTION AND DIGESTIVE DISEASES, page 890.

CITRIC ACID, a tribasic acid occurring in the juice of many fruits and in various animal tissues. It appears as translucent crystals or a white crystalline powder, soluble in water, and is employed as an acid flavoring and in effervescent drinks. Citric acid has an alkalizing effect, but is without vitamin value and is not an effective substitute for citrus fruits.

CITRIC ACID—See article CARE AND FEEDING OF THE CHILD, page 1427-28.

CLAUSTROPHOBIA, an intense fear of being in a confined area. *See also* AGORAPHOBIA.

CLAVICLE, or "collarbone," the curved bone which extends from the top of the breastbone out to each of the shoulders. Because the two clavicles are thin and small and support much weight they are frequently and easily broken. While mending, a small bony disfigurement is likely to occur, unless the person will lie motionless on his back, without a pillow, so that the two parts can remain in perfect adjustment to each other until they have completely grown together. *See also* FRACTURES.

CLEFT PALATE, a congenital defect, due to failure in fusion of embryonic facial processes, which results in a fissure through the palate. This cleavage, starting in the soft palate, may extend forward all the way across the bony roof of the mouth and even reach to the upper lip, resulting in harelip.

A person with this deformity is abnormally susceptible to inflammations in the area of the palate. Speech is difficult, as well as sucking, drinking, and chewing. Food being swallowed will frequently go through the roof of the mouth into the nostrils, and special feeding techniques become necessary.

A cleft palate can usually be corrected by an operation in which the tissues in the roof of the mouth are loosened and then fitted together. This operation is sometimes performed as early as the third month, or as late as the third year. If done before the child begins to talk, unde-

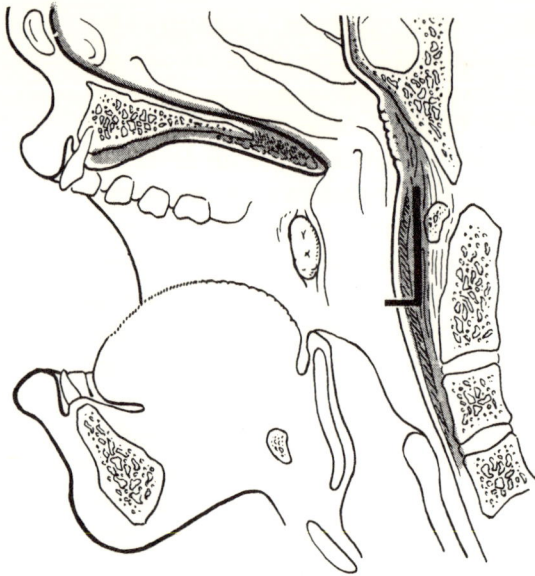

(A)

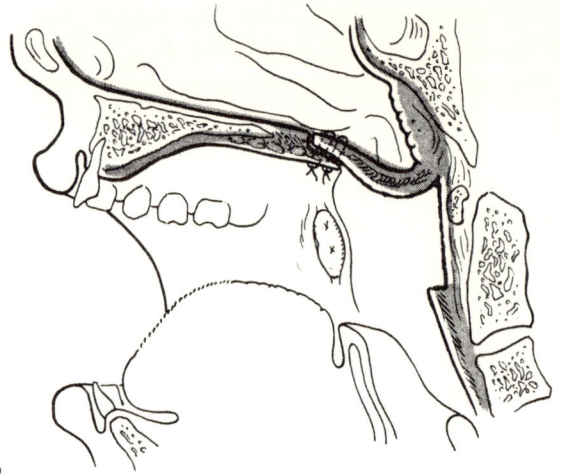

(B)

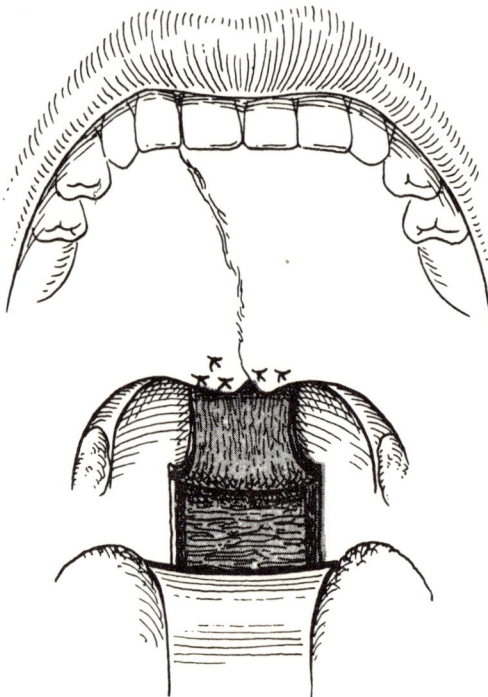

(C)

Cleft Palate — Cleft palate is the most frequent of congenital anomalies. The baby is born with a defect of the roof of the mouth. The opening in the roof of the mouth allows direct communication with the nose. Feeding is the major problem encountered with cleft palate. Sucking is difficult or impossible, and the milk tends to run out through the nose instead of being swallowed. Eventually, dentition and speech are affected. Drawing (A) shows the opening in the roof of the mouth. Part of the posterior pharyngeal flap will be brought forward and attached to the posterior end of the short soft palate. (B) shows the flap attached. (C) View of the roof of the mouth showing the repaired fissure.

sirable speech habits can be prevented. Even after a successful operation, however, some physical defect may remain. New techniques employing braces or plate or other prosthetic devices, along with intensive training, can significantly benefit persons with cleft palate. *See also* HARELIP; LIPS; PALATE.

CLIMATE, the average weather condition of an area over a period of years, as indicated by the temperature, rainfall, barometer, and other measurements. The connection between climate and health is a subject which has interested people for centuries. Greek and Roman physicians recognized that malaria affected persons living in low marshy areas, but they believed the cause of malaria was sleeping in night air. Hippocrates, the father of medicine who lived in the third century B.C., wrote, "If there be no rivers and the water that the people drink be marshy and stagnant, the physique of the people must show protruding bellies and enlarged spleens." He did not know that the protruding belly and enlarged spleen are results of malaria, prevalent in marshy areas. In his book *Air, Water and Places*, he notes that ". . . the inhabitants of a region that is mountainous, rugged, high and watered, where the changes of the seasons exhibit strong contrasts, are likely to be of big physique, with a nature well adapted for endurance and courage." This is the first recorded recognition that the Temperate Zone is a region conducive to human well-being.

More recently, persons with "consumption" or tuberculosis went to dry, high-altitude areas in an attempt to cure their illness. However, today it is felt that climate is not important in treating tuberculosis, and emphasis is placed on drugs, food, rest, and competent medical care.

Persons with rheumatic conditions frequently feel better when they are not exposed to cold and dampness. Research on rheumatism has shown that changes occur in the composition of the body tissues, including the blood, when there are changes in barometric pressure. Changes in blood supply to the joints are associated with sudden changes in temperature. While climate cannot cause rheumatic conditions, it may lower the resistance so that a rheumatic inflammation results.

For years the belief has been prevalent that dampness, cold, and drafts are associated with colds and pneumonia. However, statistics seem to indicate that, unless a person has a tendency to respiratory ailments, inclement weather does not cause such illnesses. For example, students at Stanford University at Palo Alto, California, have about as many coughs and colds as students at Harvard University in Massachusetts, despite the fact that the California climate is mild and the Massachusetts climate rigorous. However, persons whose resistance is generally low will be more susceptible to inflammation of the nose, throat, and sinuses during cold weather, and will benefit by a change to a warm dry climate.

Persons with heart disease do not do well at high altitudes, because of increased difficulty in getting oxygen for circulation.

Generally a mild climate is most beneficial to those persons with chronic diseases, and a specialist may propose that a change of climate be made to relieve their symptoms. But it is wise to check with a physician before assuming that another climate will be more beneficial.

CLIMATE — arthritis: See article ARTHRITIS, RHEUMATISM, AND GOUT, page 156-57.

CLIMATE — asthma: See article ALLERGY, page 78-79.

CLIMATE – hay fever: See article ALLERGY, page 75-76.

CLIMATE – rheumatic fever: See article DISEASES OF THE HEART AND CIRCULATION, page 1000.

CLIMATE – rheumatism: See article ARTHRITIS, RHEUMATISM, AND GOUT, page 156-57.

CLIMATE–tuberculosis: See article THE RESPIRATORY DISEASES, page 1608-10.

CLINITEST, a commercially available kit by means of which persons having or suspecting a diabetic tendency may check the extent of sugar in the urine. *See also* DIABETES.

CLITORIS, the organ in women which resembles, in miniature form, the penis of the male. This small tubelike body is located in the angle at the top of the vulva, the external sex organ of women. Like the penis, the clitoris is composed of tissue which becomes engorged with blood, and hard and erect during sexual excitement. *See also* REPRODUCTION SYSTEM.

CLITORIS – See article SEX HYGIENE, page 1671-72.

CLUBFOOT, a deformity of the foot, present at birth or caused subsequently by muscle paralysis or injury, in which the heel or the ball of the foot or one edge of it does not touch the ground.

In three-fourths of the cases noted at birth, the heel and inner edge of the foot are raised. This condition occurs once in every thousand births, and considerably more than half of those affected are male children. Also, in more than half the deformity occurs on only one side.

Treatment must be started at the earliest possible moment. The later therapy begins, the longer it will take to remedy the deformity. Children under a year can be treated in twenty-three weeks, whereas those of six years or more require almost forty-two weeks. One of the signal achievements of modern medical science has been the development of treatment for club foot.

The doctor, usually an orthopedist, will outline a routine of the manipulations of the parts involved to get them into the correct position and then make the position secure with one or more of the devices designed especially for the purpose, such as adhesive bindings, plaster casts, or braces and splints. After the proper position has been firmly established, special exercises, shoes, massage, and other measures which may be beneficial will be prescribed. Active treatment often continues for several months, and follow-up supervision is necessary for years.

Manipulation alone may not be satisfactory. Then surgical rearrangement of the affected tissues and parts becomes necessary.

The cause of clubfoot is unknown. Heredity is suspected by some persons, because approximately 5 per cent of cases occur in families in which the deformity has appeared previously; others believe that an incorrect position of the child before birth is responsible.

CLUBFOOT – See article THE FOOT, page 788-89.

COAGULATION, the formation of a coagulum, clot, or curd as in blood

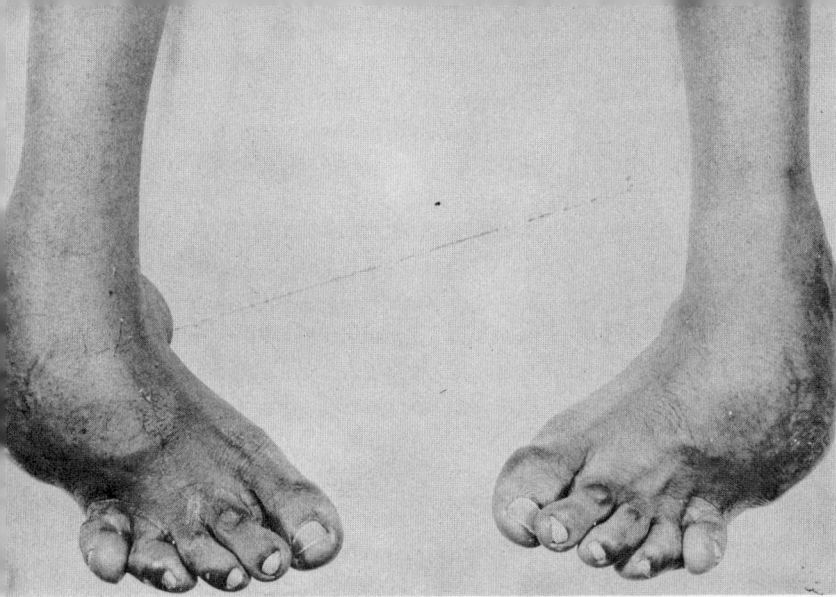

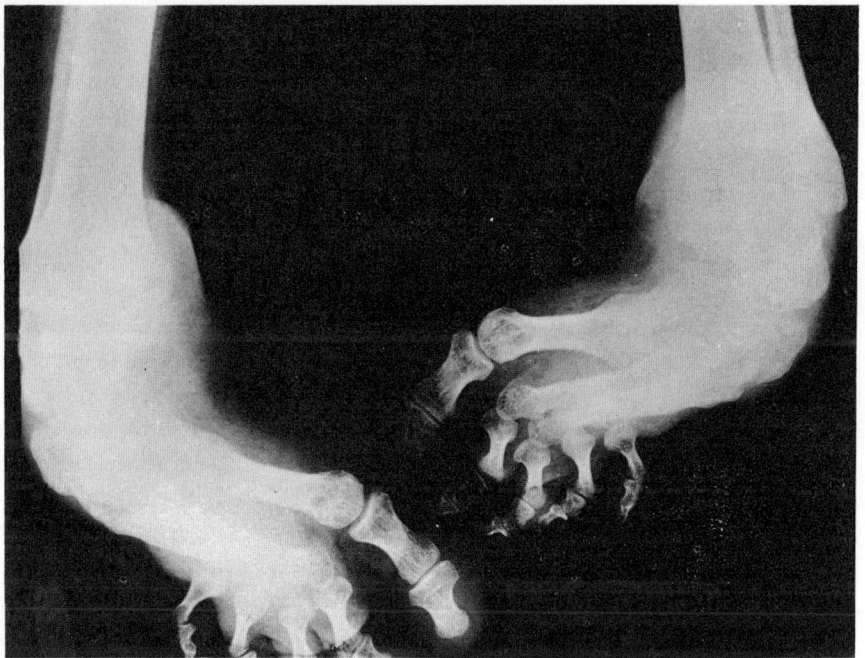

Clubfoot — Condition of clubfoot. X-ray shows the malformation of the bones in the foot. Surgery, if done early, can often correct much of the deformity in infants born with clubfoot.

or milk. When bleeding is present, threadlike fibers called fibrin are produced by a substance in the blood, the fibrinogen. These fibers trap white and red blood corpuscles which form a clot. Contraction of the fibrin squeezes out the liquid portion of the blood, the serum, and a crust develops. The system of clotting is counteracted by agents, including heparin and other anticoagulants, which keep the blood fluid. The power of coagulation of the blood varies with different persons. In people with hemophilia, a hereditary disease, the clotting is so retarded that they bleed profusely from minor wounds and may even bleed to death.

Formation of a blood clot in a coronary artery may obstruct the flow of blood to the heart muscle and produce coronary thrombosis. The incidence of clotting may be increased when the person is under stress. A blood clot blocking an artery of the brain, usually where a weak spot has resulted through arteriosclerosis, is able to produce some conditions of rheumatic heart disease. Coagulation of blood in the lower body regions can cause serious complications if particles of the blood clot reach the lungs and obstruct the major blood vessels.

In 1917, Dr. Jay McLean of Baltimore succeeded in isolating heparin, and since then dicumarol, Tromexan, and other anticoagulants have been developed and the administration of anticoagulants has become a significant medication. *See also* CORONARY THROMBOSIS; EMBOLISM; HEMOPHILIA; MENORRHAGIA.

COCAINE, an alkaloid derived from the coca bush, in use for centuries. Inca priests in Peru, for example, were aware of its anesthetic effect and chewed coca leaves in an attempt to improve their physical endurance.

Medically it was first used as an anesthetic in eye operations in Vienna in 1884. Cocaine is now employed as a local anesthetic. It produces temporary insensitivity to pain when applied to the surface of mucous membranes or injected by hypodermic needle.

Cocaine is habit-forming and poisonous, and should never be used in any way except when prescribed and administered by a physician. The amount of cocaine required to poison varies greatly; some people react unfavorably even to small doses. New synthetic compounds have been developed which are similar to cocaine but less toxic. *See also* DRUG ADDICTION.

COCAINE – poisoning: See article FIRST AID, page 831.

COCCIDIOIDOMYCOSIS, also known as desert fever, San Joaquin fever, valley fever, or the bumps, a disease with pulmonary symptoms caused by one of the fungi, coccidioides immitis, which thrives in the dry dusty areas of the San Joaquin Valley and in the southwestern states. During World War II, thousands of servicemen stationed in camps throughout this area became ill with coccidioidomycosis after inhaling the tiny invisible particles of spore-laden dust. Spores may also enter the skin through open wounds.

The first symptoms, which resemble the symptoms of tuberculosis, are generally chills, fever, headache, general malaise, night sweats, and coughing. These symptoms usually subside after a week or two and small bumps may then appear under the skin, which also disappear in time. In severe cases, x-rays show changes in the lungs and occasionally thin-walled cavities which may persist for years.

Recovery from a simple lung infection is usually rapid and complete even without treatment, but in cases where deep lung cavities have developed, surgery may be indicated.

The growing prevalence of coccidioidomycosis has made it a public health concern. About 90 per cent of the people living in these arid regions have had the infection within a ten-year period as a result of inhaling the spores of the fungus. Droughts in this area add to the disease hazards. Residents or visitors who show signs of a chronic infection resembling any of the serious respiratory diseases should have chest x-rays and skin and blood tests.

COCCYX, from the Greek meaning "shaped like the bill of a cuckoo," the last bone at the lowermost end of the spine.

CODEINE, an alkaloid derived from opium and closely allied in chemical constitution to morphine. Though weaker, its action is similar to that of morphine, and it is used medically to diminish sensitivity to pain.

CODEINE — See article DRUGS AND THEIR USES, page 616-17.
CODEINE — colds: See article THE RESPIRATORY DISEASES, page 1597.
CODEINE — shingles: See article THE SKIN, page 1763.

COD LIVER OIL, the partially destearinated fixed oil, obtained from the fresh livers of cod. The liver of the cod (and also of the halibut) is one of the richest sources of vitamin A and D, and cod liver oil has been known for many years as an effective treatment for malnutrition. Mild cases of rickets improve quickly with cod liver oil. Diets which do not contain enough fat-soluble vitamins are a basic factor of sinusitis in children, and cod liver oil is recommended by many physicians as an effective preventive measure against this infec-

tion. Every growing baby and child should have cod liver oil or its equivalent in vitamins A and D, and nursing mothers are advised by physicians to take it regularly. The amount of cod liver oil usually recommended is a teaspoonful daily of the more concentrated preparations, or two teaspoonfuls of the less concentrated. However, since today more and more foods are being vitamin-enriched, the diet usually does not need to be supplemented by cod liver oil. *See also* CHILD CARE.

COD LIVER OIL — infant's diet: See article CARE AND FEEDING OF THE CHILD, page 1429.
COD LIVER OIL — rickets: See articles CARE AND FEEDING OF THE CHILD, page 1449; DEFICIENCY DISEASES, page 508-09.
COD LIVER OIL — vitamin A: See article DEFICIENCY DISEASES, page 498-99.
COD LIVER OIL — vitamin D: See article CARE AND FEEDING OF THE CHILD, page 1419.

COFFEE, a beverage made by an infusion or decoction from the roasted and ground or pounded seeds of a shrub, small tree, or other species of the madder family. Although coffee has no nutritional value, taken in moderation it does have some distinct pharmacological worth.

In his *The Romance of Medicine,* Dr. Benjamin Lee Gordon describes its discovery. "For centuries the coffee plant was looked upon as a useless weed until one day a Turkish herdsman noticed that some goats in his charge which were feeding on the coffee beans became unusually playful and hilarious. Being curious to know the reason for their peculiar actions, he picked some coffee beans and parched them in the sun; when he reached home he brewed them and drank the beverage. To his surprise, after taking a cupful of the beverage he felt greatly stimulated without any bad effect. On the following Friday, the Mohammedan Sabbath, he treated his guests with this stimulant and they experienced the same effect. Henceforth, coffee became a national drink among Mohammedans all over the world, who use it in a strong and syrupy way."

An average cup of coffee contains about one grain of caffeine, an alkaloid which stimulates the brain, kidney, and circulation. It increases the force and beat of the heart and the flow of urine and thus helps cleanse the body of metabolic end-products. This action has made coffee valuable in cases of edema or dropsy, conditions in which fluid accumulates excessively in the tissues. In these cases, it is vital to increase the heart rate so that more blood is pumped into the blood vessels, thus promoting greater flow through the kidneys with elimination of fluid.

Generally a cup of coffee after dinner may have a good effect on the digestion since it increases the gastric juice. However, an excess of coffee can easily have toxic effects, such as rapid pulse, nervousness, irritability, and insomnia. In some persons, too much coffee may even bring on attacks of dizziness and faintness, or palpitation from an overaccelerated heart rate and force. The amount of coffee that can safely be drunk varies among people. Although Voltaire is said to have drunk more than fifty cups of coffee a day, for some people a few cups a day may be excessive.

People should discover what is the correct amount for them.

Tests made in 1955 by the American Medical Association established that a cup of regular ground coffee has almost twice as much caffeine as a cup of instant coffee, and a cup of regular decaffeinated coffee has about one-third the amount of caffeine as a cup of regular ground coffee.

COFFEE – as a stimulant: See article DRUGS AND THEIR USES, page 616-17.

COFFEE – hypertension may be aggravated by: See article BLOOD PRESSURE, pages 254, 256, 258.

COLCHICINE, a water-soluble, pale brownish alkaloid derived from the meadow saffron which has been used as an efficient pain reliever in gout for more than a hundred years. However, it has proved of little value in other types of arthritis and rheumatism. *See also* GOUT.

COLCHICINE – See article ARTHRITIS, RHEUMATISM, AND GOUT, page 162-63.

COLD. *See* COMMON COLD.

COLD CREAM, a mixture in an ointment of petrolatum, lanolin, and rosewater, which is useful for soothing dry, inflamed, or irritated skin, and also for removing cosmetics. *See also* COSMETICS.

COLD CREAM – medicine chest: See article THE FAMILY MEDICINE CHEST, page 1254-55.

COLD CREAM – senile freckles: See article THE SKIN, page 1778.

COLD CREAM – skin care: See article THE SKIN, pages 1736, 1738.

COLD CREAM – soap substitute: See article THE SKIN, page 1728.

COLD CREAM – sunburn: See article THE SKIN, pages 1750, 1755.

446

fuse lupus erythematosus, scleroderma, and dermatomyositis. They resemble each other in that all of them represent disturbances of connective tissue in the body in contrast to glandular tissue or surface secreting tissue. An important fact about the collagen diseases is the discovery, made in 1950, that all of them are benefited, at least temporarily, by ACTH or cortisone. Arthritis, which also responds to the drugs mentioned, occurs commonly in connection with each of these diseases.

Polyarteritis nodosa. Polyarteritis nodosa is a disease in which the blood vessels are chiefly affected. Only about 500 cases of this disease have been reported. Because this disease is primarily associated with serious damage of blood vessels, it may occur in any part of the body. The condition affects men four times as often as women and mostly those between twenty and forty years old. Arthritis and many of the reactions associated with hypersensitivity are observed in this disease.

Lupus erythematosus. Disseminated lupus erythematosus is a chronic, usually severe, disorder occurring mostly in females fifteen to forty years old. A characteristic is a butterfly-shaped inflammation over the nose. Other symptoms involve the joints and the heart.

Scleroderma. Scleroderma is a disease that affects the connective tissue of the body and particularly that in the skin, where there is hardening. Chiefly women between thirty and fifty years old are affected. The swelling in the skin may be followed by calcification. This disease comes on slowly and insidiously, but as it progresses, changes occur in the skin of the face, neck and arms. The skin looks waxy and tight and loses its color and hair. When the face is involved there may be difficulty in moving the jaw. Fortunately this is not a common disease; certainly it is not as serious as polyarteritis nodosa or diffuse lupus erythematosus, which are similar. In the older forms of treatment emphasis was placed on the use of thyroid and vitamins. Great care was given to prevent secondary infections. More recently attention is being focused on the use of ACTH and cortisone.

Dermatomyositis. Fourth in this group of collagen disorders is one called dermatomyositis. This is a common and often fatal disorder involving the skin and the muscles. The exact cause is still unknown. It affects people of all races and colors, both men and women, and in general those between the ages of ten and fifty years.

Characteristic of this condition is the involvement of the muscles. As they deteriorate, the organs concerned show effects, as in the eyes, throat, diaphragm, or muscles between the ribs. The symptoms then are difficulties of vision, swallowing, breathing, speech, etc. These symptoms are accompanied by weakness and loss of weight.

COLLAGEN DISEASES – See article DIS-EASES OF THE HEART AND CIRCULATION, page 998.

COLLARBONE, the common name for clavicle. *See also* CLAVICLE.

COLLODION, a coating or film used to protect and dress wounds. It is produced by dissolving gun cotton in ether and alcohol.

COLOSTOMY, a surgical operation, usually on the left side of the lower abdomen, creating a more or less permanent opening in the colon to permit evacuation after the normal rectal and anal opening is lost.

COLOSTOMY — See article DIGESTION AND DIGESTIVE DISEASES, page 901.

COMA, a state of complete loss of consciousness from which the person cannot be aroused even by the most powerful stimulation. The forms of coma most frequently seen are those following alcoholic intoxication and that which occurs in diabetes. The treatment of such forms of coma is so serious that it should never be undertaken except by a physician. *See also* DIABETES.

COMA — diabetic: See article DIABETES, page 583-86.

COMMON COLD, an acute inflammation of the upper respiratory tract, involving the nose and throat. It is one of the most familiar ailments which afflicts mankind yet its specific cause is little understood. Susceptibility to colds is almost universal,

Causes of coma in a large city hospital   100%

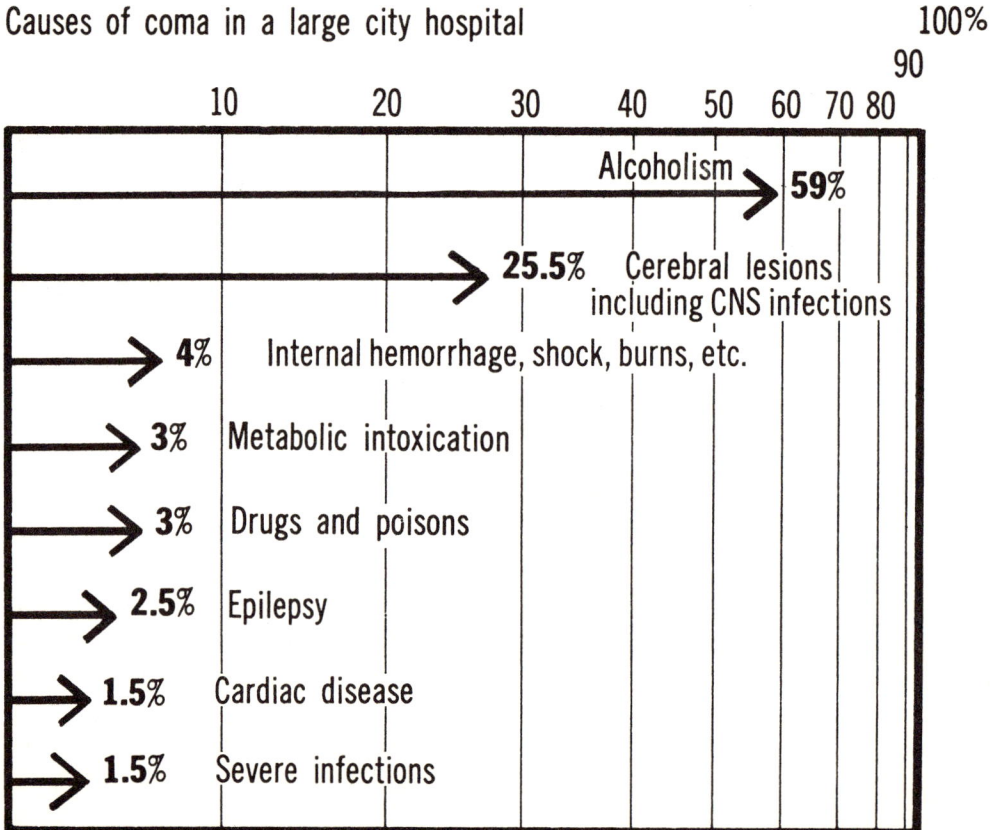

Causes of coma in a large city hospital

- Alcoholism → **59%**
- 25.5% Cerebral lesions including CNS infections
- 4% Internal hemorrhage, shock, burns, etc.
- 3% Metabolic intoxication
- 3% Drugs and poisons
- 2.5% Epilepsy
- 1.5% Cardiac disease
- 1.5% Severe infections

(Scale: 10 20 30 40 50 60 70 80 90 100%)

particularly among children. The cold is highly contagious, especially indoors, and places where groups of people congregate are excellent transmission spots for the infection.

In large urban communities where the climate is temperate, the general population averages about three colds a year. This median is higher among susceptible adults and children. The incidence is lowest in the summer, rises in the autumn, reaching its peak in midwinter and declines in the spring.

Several peak periods occur in smaller urban communities. The first is in early autumn when schools reopen and children are brought into greater proximity indoors. In addition to the winter rise in incidence of colds, a smaller rise often appears in the spring.

Colds are definitely communicable and are transmitted either by direct contact or by spread of the infected droplets of discharge. A practical method to control the spread of colds has not yet been developed. The common cold is due to one or more viruses. Scientists believe that the virus is generally present in the throat but it becomes active only when the body resistance is lowered. When the cold virus attacks the mucous membranes of the nose and throat, these tissues are weakened and become susceptible to infection by bacteria which are also generally found in the body. The bacteria are secondary invaders and the virus paves the way for their entry into the mucous membranes. Although they are not responsible for the common cold, the bacteria

may initiate a secondary infection which either intensifies the local inflammation present, prolonging the cold, or causes new complications such as purulent sinusitis or otitis, an inflammation of the ear. Infants and young children appear to be more susceptible to these secondary infections than adults.

A cold usually begins abruptly, with a sense of soreness and dryness in the nose or back of the throat. Within a few hours the nasal passages feel congested, sneezing develops and a colorless watery discharge comes from the nose. After forty-eight hours the cold is usually at its peak, and is accompanied by excessive watering of the eyes, huskiness of the voice, and difficulty in breathing as the congestion spreads. The nasal discharge becomes thick and sticky and some coughing may develop. The cough does not usually bring up much discharge unless the person has a tendency to chronic bronchitis. Frequently a headache, a sense of lethargy and malaise, and vague pains in the back and limbs accompany a cold. A fever is rarely present, although in children a temperature of 102° or even higher often develops.

The uncomplicated cold generally lasts from one to two weeks and terminates without special treatment. Colds which persist or recur repeatedly, or in which there is a steady prolonged fever or chills, particularly in children or susceptible adults, may indicate complications and a physician should be consulted. As yet, a specific agent has not been developed to control the common cold and treatment is confined to relief of symptoms and control of complications. Treatment of the cold is not very different today from the treatment used by past generations. Bed rest should be enforced whenever possible and as much isolation as is practical. Plenty of liquids, hot or cold, a light diet, and keeping warm promote greater comfort. Aspirin in small repeated doses generally gives relief as does gargling in cases of sore throat. An aspirin tablet or a teaspoon of salt dissolved in hot water is beneficial. In the latter stages of a cold, when the discharge has thickened, an atomizer or nose drops or inhaler helps clear the nasal passages. They should not be used more than once in four hours and if the person has a tendency to nasal inflammation should be employed sparingly.

Cold vaccines, which are suspensions of dead bacteria collected from the discharge of a cold, have not been found to be significantly effective either when taken by mouth or when given as an injection or nasal spray. However, continued research is being done. The routine use of sulfonamides or antibiotics for colds is definitely discouraged. These drugs should be given only in cases with a definite bacterial secondary infection —for example, in bronchopneumonia, sinusitis, or otitis media. Persons who have a consistent history of recurrent colds with accompanying complications may use antibiotics or sulfonamides, but only on the advice of a physician.

Although little is known about curing a cold, measures can be taken to ward off the infection and decrease its incidence. A well-balanced diet, sufficient rest, proper dress both indoors and out, all help to keep the body resistance high. Undue exposure to sharp changes in temperature should be avoided. Proper ventilation of rooms, with sufficient humidity in the air, helps to keep the mucous membranes in healthy condition. If humidifiers are not used, adequate moisture can be maintained by keeping a pan of water on a radiator or stove. Particular care should be taken to avoid contact with persons who have colds. Simple hygienic measures like washing the hands before eating or covering a sneeze all help to decrease the occurrence of colds. *See also* BRONCHOPNEUMONIA; CHILD CARE; OTITIS; SINUSES.

COMMON COLD – infants: See article CARE AND FEEDING OF THE CHILD, page 1431.

COMMON COLD – nasal allergy confused with: See article ALLERGY, pages 76,78.

COMMON COLD – prevention: See article THE RESPIRATORY DISEASES, page 1590-97.

COMMON COLD – respiratory disease: See article THE RESPIRATORY DISEASES, page 1599-1603.

COMMON COLD – rheumatic fever may recur after: See article DISEASES OF THE HEART AND CIRCULATION, page 987.

COMMON COLD – rose: See article THE RESPIRATORY DISEASES, page 1598.

COMMON COLD – spring: See article THE RESPIRATORY DISEASES, page 1598.

COMMON COLD – summer: See article THE RESPIRATORY DISEASES, page 1598.

COMMON COLD – symptoms: See article THE RESPIRATORY DISEASES, pages 1590, 1592.

COMMON COLD–treatment: See article THE RESPIRATORY DISEASES, page 1596-98.

COMMON COLD – undulant fever mistaken for: See article TRANSMISSIBLE DISEASES, page 1905.

COMMON COLD – vaccines: See article THE REPIRATORY DISEASES, pages 1594, 1596-97.

COMMON COLD – whooping cough resembles: See article INFECTIOUS DISEASES OF CHILDHOOD, page 1114-15.

COMMUNICABLE DISEASES, those which are transmissible from one person to another. The difference, often disregarded, between infectious and communicable contagious diseases is that while infectious diseases are caused by the invasion of an infective agent like a fungus bacillus, or virus, the agents are not necessarily transmitted by a person.

COMMUNICABLE DISEASES – SEE INFECTIOUS DISEASES.

COMPOUND FRACTURE. The breaking of a bone is a fracture. In a compound fracture, the point of the fracture is in contact with the outer surface of the body—for example, through a wound. If the break is covered by the skin, it is a simple fracture. *See also* BONES; FIRST AID; FRACTURES.

COMPRESS, a piece of folded gauze, cloth, or a soft pad which is applied firmly to a part of the body to relieve inflammations, produce pressure, or prevent hemorrhage. It may be wet or dry, hot or cold, and is sometimes perforated for drainage or observation of the underlying skin.

COMPULSION, defined in psychology as an irresistible, irrational desire to repeat certain acts. For example, a person may have the compulsion to wash his hands every few minutes, or to avoid stepping on the cracks in the sidewalk.

CONCEPTION, the union of sperm and ovum, the male and female sex cells, leading to the development of a new life. Conception is sometimes called fertilization, impregnation, or fecundation, and should be distinguished from the term copulation which refers to the act of sexual union between the male and female.

Since the egg cell of the female lives for only about twelve hours out of every month, the male seed must be deposited within the female genital tract during these few hours, or within two or three days of release of an egg. The sperm cells live about three days after ejaculation.

Conception usually takes place within the Fallopian tubes adjacent to the uterus and ovaries, and may occur within an hour of intercourse. Following union of the male and female sex cells, development is rapid, and eight to fourteen days later the product imbeds itself in the lining of the uterus where it remains until birth. *See also* REPRODUCTION SYSTEM.

CONCEPTION – prevention of: SEE CONTRACEPTION.

CONCUSSION, a shock, severe shaking or jarring of a part of the body, usually resulting from a fall or blow. It also refers to the morbid state resulting from such a jarring. A concussion of the brain is actually a paralysis of its function, and symptoms are not due to any fracture or laceration. Signs of hemorrhage or loss of blood from the coverings around the brain may be present. Sometimes disturbances occur in the circulation of spinal fluid through the brain, and occasionally part of the soft white material of the brain is crushed or the connection cords between different portions of the brain are damaged or destroyed.

Brain concussion itself is seldom fatal. Necropsies (post-mortems) have shown that some apparent serious lesion of brain substance or vessels has occurred in fatal cases which had the characteristics of concussion but actually were contusions or lacerations. Whenever a concussion is suspected, a physician should be consulted. An x-ray examination should be made to determine whether or not fracture of the skull or other complications have occurred. While a slight crack of the skull is

not critical, the pressure that may result from the bleeding inside the skull may be.

Symptoms of concussion appear immediately after the injury and vary depending on the degree of injury. Probably there will be a severe aching of the head, a weak dizzy "stunned" feeling. Disturbances in vision, cold perspiration, and shallow respiration may appear. If the jarring has been severe, more extreme symptoms may develop at once. The victim may be in partial coma or unconscious. The body will be cold and respiration exceedingly weak. Often vomiting accompanies these symptoms.

The consequences of a concussion may be of short duration or last for days or weeks or longer. Often, after regaining his senses, the person is unable to remember anything that happened during the time when consciousness was lost. Frequently symptoms of contusion and hemorrhage may develop and with them serious brain injuries. When the symptoms are protracted, a more serious affliction is always suggested.

During emergency treatment, the person should lie flat and be kept warm and quiet. Attempts at stimulation should not be made. No pressure should be applied or strong antiseptics given. *See also* HEAD INJURIES; SHOCK.

CONDITIONING, the development of a better physiological condition through physical exercise and training.

A great football coach once said

vary from few or none at all to a condition resembling a wasting disease. Loss of appetite comes early and halitosis is likely. The person becomes depressed and dull without apparent cause, tires easily, cannot cope with his responsibilities as usual, and may look pale and unwell. Frequent indigestion and discomfort or pain in the digestive system are common.

The doctor can establish whether bad habits and overdosing with purgatives are responsible, or whether deep-seated organic disorders may be present. In any event, only the doctor can safely outline the measures to be followed.

In most cases of dyschesia, or constipation involving largely the lower end of the digestive tract, actual re-education is necessary to start regularity and reliance on natural processes. Often, however, enemas, suppositories, or mild laxatives may be used to get new habits under way. Regular exercise is frequently advisable, especially for a sedentary person. A walk before breakfast or daily exercise of the abdominal muscles may be desirable.

Along with re-education, an adequately varied diet is probably more significant than any other factor. The major constituents of a normal diet, proteins, carbohydrates, fats, mineral salts, vitamins, and sufficient indigestible bulk, should all be assured. Fruit, especially stewed prunes and apples, are recommended for breakfast, and green vegetables and salad at both luncheon and the evening meal. Bran should be considered as a medicinal food, to be used only on the physician's advice, because it seems to accomplish little more than other bulk foods and may be irritating to the bowel.

Many drugs are available for treating various kinds of constipation. Vegetable and salt cathartics, organic and mineral medicines, substances which act mechanically, and water in various forms are among the most common. Cathartics of both the mineral and vegetable types irritate the bowel and are not advised for long use. They include the strong salts, cascara, jalap, senna, rhubarb, and aloes. Among the substances that act mechanically are mineral oil, bran, agar-agar, flax seeds, and psyllium seeds which lubricate the digestive tract or work by pushing its contents before them. Mixtures of mineral oil and such materials as agar-agar or flax seeds form a mucilaginous mass. Caution is necessary in using mineral oil because it absorbs vitamin A and may lead to a deficiency of that vitamin, and also because of a tendency of mineral oil to leak out of the bowel. Phenolphthalein is the chief ingredient of many widely used laxative combinations.

Recently attention has been given to methods of assisting the body itself to prevent overdryness of the bowel. If the amount of bile discharged by the liver is increased, making it thinner and greater in volume, the contents of the bowel remain softer and evacuation is easier and more normal when there has previously been a difficulty with overdry elimination. Bile acids have been found to accomplish this better than bile salts, which doctors formerly gave, because they thin the bile in the liver and enable it to be secreted more profusely. This is a normal body process and advantageous when constipation must be treated.

More than $50,000,000 a year is spent in the United States on constipation remedies. Cathartics, when taken habitually, end by defeating their purpose and may make elimination more difficult rather than less difficult. Some have a useful function, but they are best prescribed by a doctor.

CONTACT DERMATITIS, an inflammation of the skin due to a sensitization to a substance with which it comes in contact. As a permanent injury to health, contact dermatitis is not a serious disturbance, but this minor allergy is persistent and often exceedingly annoying. It affects all age groups from infants to old people.

Whenever the skin is exposed to allergens, substances to which a person is sensitive, rashes, hives, cracks, burning, sores, and other irritations may develop. A good example is poison ivy in which an itchy rash is produced on the skin through contact with an oil in the poison ivy plant.

The substances to which a sensitive person may react on touch are numerous and include plants, wood, fur, silk, wool, dye, resin, plastic, rubber, metal, and many more. Some women have cosmetic contact dermatitis and cannot use ordinary beauty products such as soap, bleaches, deodorants, or powder. The active reaction of the skin to an allergenic substance makes contact dermatitis an occupational disorder too, and it frequently affects industrial workers who are exposed to certain chemicals, wood, metal, glue, or lacquer. In some instances, skin disorders spread to the nail bed and produce a condition called onycholysis. Nails may become brittle, separate into layers, or fall out completely.

Where factory workers are sensitive to given substances, preventive steps must be taken. Forced circulation of air, which removes dust to which a person may be sensitive, is one such preventive measure. Compulsory showers, protective clothing, face respirators and gloves are other measures.

When symptoms of contact dermatitis apear, the cause should be determined. A physician may discover the source through a patch test as in other allergies and then proceed with special desensitization which is possible with a number of materials.

CONTACT DERMATITIS — See article AL-LERGY, page 82-84.

CONTACT DERMATITIS — scalp: See article THE HAIR, page 953.

CONTACT LENSES, eyeglasses that fit directly over the eyeball and fully aid the vision. A mold of the eye is made, exactly as one makes a cast of the inside of the mouth when it is necessary to have false teeth on plates. From this fragile mold a permanent one is made with dental plastic; then the glass is modeled to fit the mold. The inner surface of the contact lens must fit the eyeball so that it will not injure the sensitive tissues or interfere with the circulation of the blood. Before the mold has been prepared, it is necessary to fit the contact lenses. This means that the eye must be studied by all of the usual methods in order to determine the difficulties of vision so that the lens will meet its needs.

The fitting of contact lenses is a procedure performed by experts in ophthalmology or optometry with the aid of the optician. In fitting the lens, the lids of the eye are separated by the thumb and forefinger of the left hand and the contact lens is then inserted between the eyelids and the eyeball, usually first beneath the lower eyelid and then beneath the upper. Special fluids are used in preparing the eye for the lens and for helping the eye to become accustomed to its use. Preferably the contact lens must fit closely and any bubbles of fluid must be removed before it is considered in suitable position. Once the lens is fitted correctly, the wearer must practice setting and removing the contact lens so that the placing of the lens and its retention become a habit. In developing this procedure, the optician who fits the lens is helpful in observing the practice until it becomes perfect.

Experiments have shown that the average person learns to insert the lenses in approximately nine minutes. At first, these lenses are worn only an hour or two at a time, but many who become well accustomed to them wear their lenses six to eight hours. Several months may be required, in some cases, before the person becomes sufficiently used to contact lenses to be able to wear them a long time without removing them and refilling them with fluid, and also without resting the eyes.

CONTRACEPTION, the use of a device, substance, or method to prevent conception during sexual intercourse.

Perhaps the commonest of the various methods of contraception are the use of the sheath or condom of rubber worn by the man and, alternatively, the pessary or diaphragm worn by the woman. Chemicals, especially fixed in thick creams, which destroy or immobilize the sperm cell are also used. The American Medical Association has listed a number of such creams by name, as acceptable when prescribed by the doctor.

The physician's advice as to the proper use of such devices, materials, and methods is desirable, since not all are of equal effectiveness. The combination of pessary and cream, for instance, is probably 90 per cent or more effective; none is 100 per cent reliable. The pessary must be prescribed and fitted for the woman by the physician; otherwise, at best, its use will be haphazard protection. Creams and other chemicals are safe only on the advice of a physician. The use of douches is also common, but if they are to be effective and safe, should be employed only with medical advice. Many cleansing or sterilizing agents are dangerous to the body, or may alter normal bacterial growth undesirably in the parts where they are used.

Another method of avoiding conception is the so-called rhythm technique. The basis for this theory is the regular monthly cycle of ovulation. An egg cell or ovum passes from the ovary once every month, and consequently during the month the woman is more likely to conceive at one time than another. These intervals are commonly referred to respectively as the fertile and the safe periods. For the woman who menstruates regularly every twenty-eight days, the safe period is calculated as approximately a week before and a week after menstruation. More exactly, it lasts nine days, beginning the first day of menstruation. The fertile period, which normally is a maximum of eight days, follows, and then the next eleven days are again "safe." When the menstrual interval is shorter or longer than this, or is irregular, the physician's advice is desirable.

Another way of identifying the fertile period is to record the morning temperature, before any food is eaten or water or other fluids are drunk. Ovulation brings with it a fall in temperature, then a rise. Abstinence is practiced during the period of ovulation, and for three days before and three days after.

The latest development is a pill of progestin called Enovid and Orthonovum which prohibits ovulation. Five days after cessation of menstruation a pill is taken daily for twenty days. The products are also useful in various menstrual disturbances.

CONTRACEPTION — arrangement during early days of marriage: See article SEX HYGIENE, page 1693-94.

CONTRACEPTION—dangers: See article SEX HYGIENE, page 1705.

CONTRACEPTION — drugs: See article DRUGS AND THEIR USES, page 616-17.

CONTUSION, a superficial injury or bruise, produced by impact, in which breaking of the skin does not occur. If the skin is punctured also, the term contused wound is used. *See also* BRUISES.

CONTUSION — See article DISEASES OF THE HEART AND CIRCULATION, page 983-84.

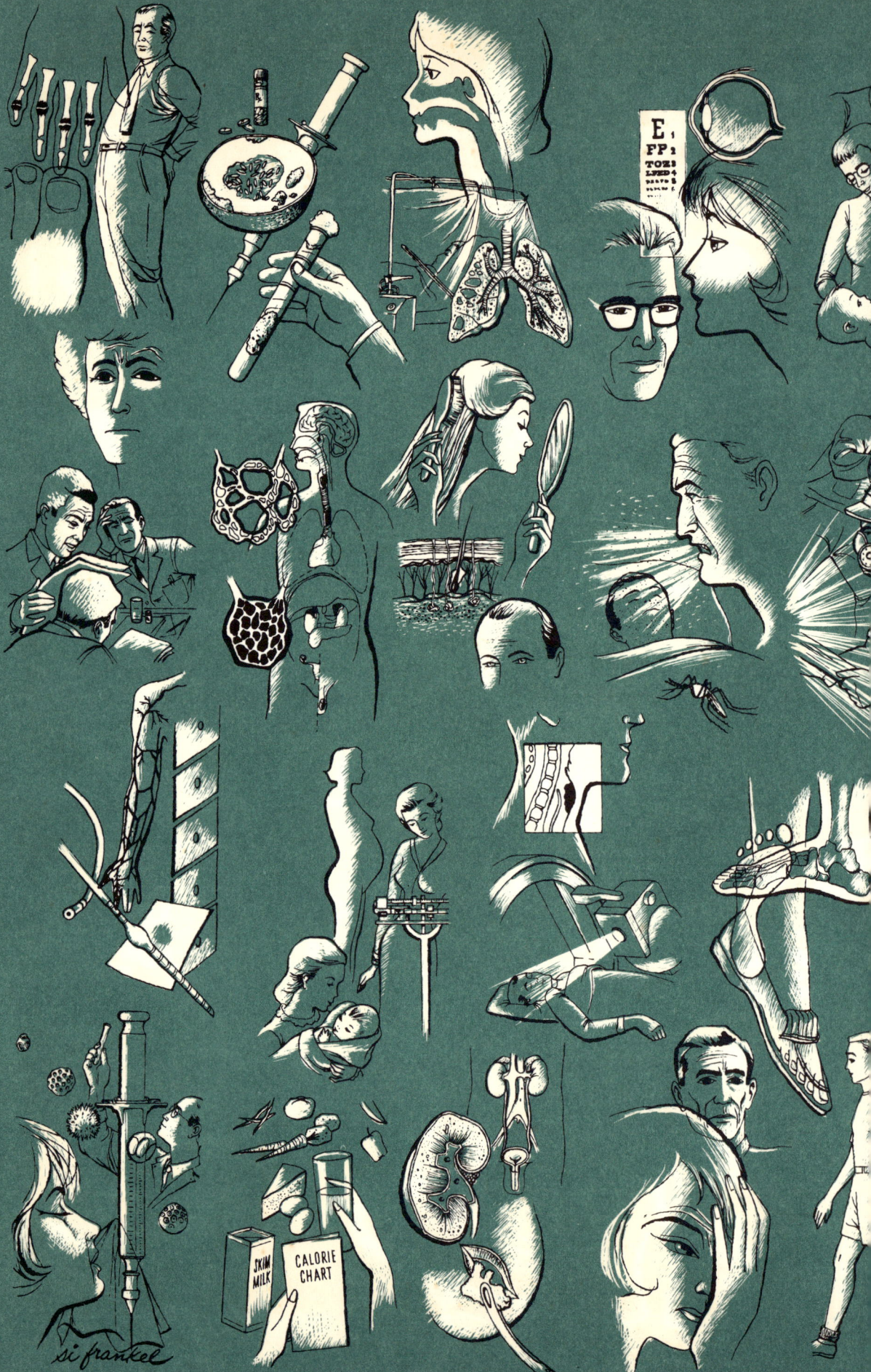

si frankel